INTRODUCTION TO

Physical Therapy

for

Physical Therapist Assistants

Olga Dreeben, PT, PhD, MPT
Director and Professor
Physical Therapist Assistant Program
Lake City Community College
Lake City, Florida

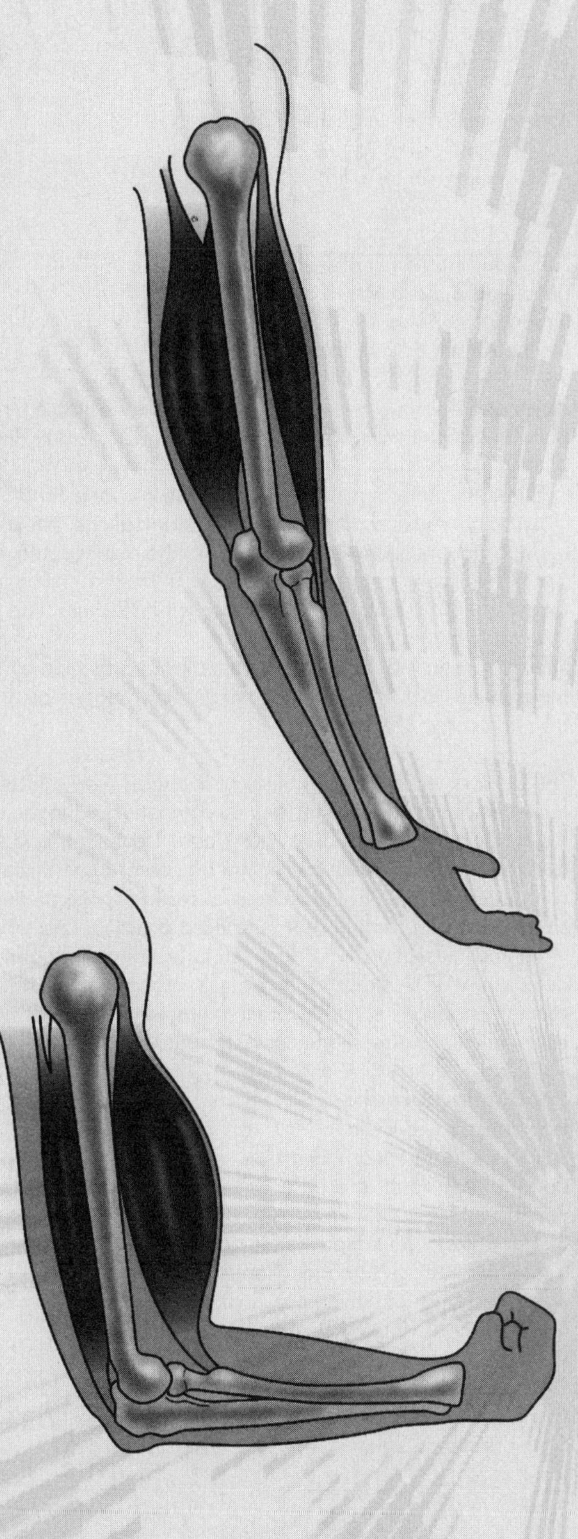

JONES AND BARTLETT PUBLISHERS

Sudbury, Massachusetts

BOSTON   TORONTO   LONDON   SINGAPORE

World Headquarters
Jones and Bartlett Publishers
40 Tall Pine Drive
Sudbury, MA 01776
978-443-5000
info@jbpub.com
www.jbpub.com

Jones and Bartlett Publishers Canada
6339 Ormindale Way
Mississauga, Ontario L5V 1J2
Canada

Jones and Bartlett Publishers International
Barb House, Barb Mews
London W6 7PA
United Kingdom

Jones and Bartlett's books and products are available through most bookstores and online booksellers. To contact Jones and Bartlett Publishers directly, call 800-832-0034, fax 978-443-8000, or visit our website www.jbpub.com.

Substantial discounts on bulk quantities of Jones and Bartlett's publications are available to corporations, professional associations, and other qualified organizations. For details and specific discount information, contact the special sales department at Jones and Bartlett via the above contact information or send an email to specialsales@jbpub.com.

The authors, editor, and publisher have made every effort to provide accurate information. However, they are not responsible for errors, omissions, or for any outcomes related to the use of the contents of this book and take no responsibility for the use of the products and procedures described. Treatments and side effects described in this book may not be applicable to all people; likewise, some people may require a dose or experience a side effect that is not described herein. Drugs and medical devices are discussed that may have limited availability controlled by the Food and Drug Administration (FDA) for use only in a research study or clinical trial. Research, clinical practice, and government regulations often change the accepted standard in this field. When consideration is being given to use of any drug in the clinical setting, the health care provider or reader is responsible for determining FDA status of the drug, reading the package insert, and reviewing prescribing information for the most up-to-date recommendations on dose, precautions, and contraindications, and determining the appropriate usage for the product. This is especially important in the case of drugs that are new or seldom used.

Production Credits
Publisher: David Cella
Associate Editor: Maro Gartside
Editorial Assistant: Teresa Reilly
Production Director: Amy Rose
Senior Production Editor: Renée Sekerak
Senior Marketing Manager: Sophie Fleck
Manufacturing and Inventory Control Supervisor: Amy Bacus
Cover Design: Timothy Dziewit
Composition: John Garland
Cover Background Image: © †ELEN/ShutterStock, Inc.
Printing and Binding: Courier
Cover Printing: Courier

ISBN: 978-0-7637-7953-5

6048
Printed in the United States of America
13 12 11 10 09   10 9 8 7 6 5 4 3 2

Contents

How This Book Can Help You Learn

All of us have different learning styles. Some of us are visual learners, some more auditory, some learn better by doing an activity. Some students prefer to learn new material using visual aids. Some learn material better when they hear it in a lecture; others learn it better by reading it. Cognitive research has shown that no matter what your learning style, you will learn more if you are actively engaged in the learning process.

This Student Study Guide will help you learn by providing a structure to your notes and letting you utilize all of the learning styles mentioned above. Students don't need to copy down every word their professor says or recopy their entire textbook. Do the assigned reading, listen in lecture, follow the key points your instructor is making, and write down meaningful notes. After reading and lectures, review your notes and pull out the most important points.

The Student Study Guide is your partner and guide in note-taking. Your Guide provides you with a visual guide that follows the chapter topics presented in your textbook. If your instructor is using the PowerPoint slides that accompany the text, this guide will save you from having to write down everything that is on the slides. There is space provided for you to jot down the terms and concepts that you feel are most important to each lecture. By working with your Guide, you are seeing, hearing, writing, and, later, reading and reviewing. The more often you are exposed to the material, the better you will learn and understand it. Using different methods of exposure significantly increases your comprehension.

Your Guide is the perfect place to write down questions that you want to ask your professor later, interesting ideas that you want to discuss with your study group, or reminders to yourself to go back and study a certain concept again to make sure that you really got it.

Having organized notes is essential at exam time and when doing homework assignments. Your ability to easily locate the important concepts of a recent lecture will help you move along more rapidly, as you don't have to spend time rereading an entire chapter just to reinforce one point that you may not have quite understood.

Your Guide is a valuable resource. You've found a wonderful study partner!

Note-Taking Tips

1. It is easier to take notes if you are not hearing the information for the first time. Read the chapter or the material that is about to be discussed before class. This will help you to anticipate what will be said in class, and have an idea of what to write down. It will also help to read over your notes from the last class. This way you can avoid having to spend the first few minutes of class trying to remember where you left off last time.

2. Don't waste your time trying to write down everything that your professor says. Instead, listen closely and only write down the important points. Review these important points after class to help remind you of related points that were made during the lecture.

3. If the class discussion takes a spontaneous turn, pay attention and participate in the discussion. Only take notes on the conclusions that are relevant to the lecture.

4. Emphasize main points in your notes. You may want to use a highlighter, special notation (asterisks, exclamation points), format (circle, underline), or placement on the page (indented, bulleted). You will find that when you try to recall these points, you will be able to actually picture them on the page.

5. Be sure to copy down word-for-word specific formulas, laws, and theories.

6. Hearing something repeated, stressed, or summed up can be a signal that it is an important concept to understand.

7. Organize handouts, study guides, and exams in your notebook along with your lecture notes. It may be helpful to use a three-ring binder, so that you can insert pages wherever you need to.

8. When taking notes, you might find it helpful to leave a wide margin on all four sides of the page. Doing this allows you to note names, dates, definitions, etc., for easy access and studying later. It may also be helpful to make notes of questions you want to ask your professor about or research later, ideas or relationships that you want to explore more on your own, or concepts that you don't fully understand.

9. It is best to maintain a separate notebook for each class. Labeling and dating your notes can be helpful when you need to look up information from previous lectures.

10. Make your notes legible, and take notes directly in your notebook. Chances are you won't recopy them no matter how noble your intentions. Spend the time you would have spent recopying the notes studying them instead, drawing conclusions and making connections that you didn't have time for in class.

11. Look over your notes after class while the lecture is still fresh in your mind. Fix illegible items and clarify anything you don't understand. Do this again right before the next class.

THE PROFESSION OF PHYSICAL THERAPY

INTRODUCTION TO PART I

Part I of this textbook, called "The Profession of Physical Therapy," is divided in two chapters:

- Chapter 1: Development of the Physical Therapy Profession
- Chapter 2: The Physical Therapist Assistant as a Member of the Health Care Team

In these two chapters, we will discuss the history of rehabilitation treatments including therapeutic exercises and the organization, history, values, and the culture of the profession of physical therapy. We will also explore the differences in role, function, and supervisory relationship of the physical therapist (PT), the physical therapist assistant (PTA), and other health care practitioners and ancillary personnel.

LABORATORY ACTIVITIES FOR PART I

The following activities are suggested to the instructor to involve students in the application of laboratory performances:

- Go online at www.apta.org/rt.cfm/About and research information about the APTA.
- Create a brochure identifying the vision, mission, and function of the APTA and the benefits of belonging to the APTA.
- Participate in a district or chapter/subchapter meeting.
- Create a class presentation about what PTAs are and what they do.
- Interview a health care professional, such as a PT, OT, SLP or SW. Create a class presentation about the function, role, and interaction of the health care professional.
- Make a list of terminology found in the Guide related to physical therapy interventions.
- Interview a classmate or be interviewed by a classmate.
- Write a resume.
- Write at least one policy and one procedure.

Development of the Physical Therapy Profession

After studying Chapter 1, the reader will be able to:

- Discuss the history of rehabilitation treatments (including therapeutic exercises) from ancient times through the 1900s.
- Describe the history of the physical therapy profession and its five cycles of growth and development.
- Understand the values and culture of the physical therapy profession.
- Consider the American Physical Therapy Association's mission and its goals (especially goals two and six) in regard to physical therapists and physical therapist assistants.
- Explain the organizational structure of the American Physical Therapy Association.
- Discuss the benefits of belonging to a professional organization.
- Name the other organizations involved in the physical therapy profession.

GLOSSARY

Disability: The inability to engage in age-specific, gender-related, and sex-specific roles in a particular social context and physical environment; it is also any restriction or lack (resulting from an injury) of ability to perform an activity in a manner or within the range considered normal for a human being.

Dislocation: Temporary displacement of the bone from its normal position in a joint; occurs with tearing of ligaments, tendons, and articular capsules.

Electrotherapy: The use of electrical stimulation modalities in physical therapy treatment.

Hydrotherapy: Physical therapy intervention using water.

Proprioceptive neuromuscular facilitation (PNF): A form of therapeutic exercise in which accommodating resistance Is manually applied to various patterns of movement for the purpose of strengthening the muscles.

Notes

CHAPTER 1

DEVELOPMENT OF THE PHYSICAL THERAPY PROFESSION

History of Rehabilitation Treatments

- 3000BC: China–therapeutic ex., massage, hydrotherapy
- 1000BC: China-Cong Fu ex.
- 500BC: Herodicus–Ars Gymnastica
- 400BC: Hippocrates–muscle strength
- 180BC: Ancient Rome–gymnastics
- 2nd century AD: Galen–moderate ex.
- 1735: Europe–ex. equipment
- Per Henrik Ling: Swedish Gymnastics and Massage

History of Rehabilitation Treatments

- 1864: Gustav Zander–machines
- 1860: electrical stimulation
- 1890: Nikola Tesla–diathermy
- Proprioceptive facilitation: Kabat
- 1889: Frenkel–sensory deficits ex.
- Lovett: polio muscle training
- Wright: gait training (crutches) and MMT
- Hydrotherapy: Lowman and Hubbard
- Exercises: Buerger, Williams, Codman, DeLorme (PREs)
- Isokinetic: Hislop and Perrine

History of the Physical Therapy Profession

Formative Year: 1914–1920

- Division of Special Hospitals and Physical Reconstruction–1917
- Reconstruction Therapy–rehabilitation program–World War I soldiers
- Physical therapy units–1917: gymnasium, whirlpool, massage/mechanotherapy rooms
- Reconstruction Aides–PT/OT pioneers
- Mary McMillan trained Reconstruction Aides–Reed College, Portland, Oregon–1918
- Mary McMillan–Walter Reed Hospital–1919

History of the Physical Therapy Profession

Development Years: 1920–1940

- American Women's Physical Therapeutics (AWPT): January 1921
- Mary McMillan: AWPT President–1921–1923
- P.T. Review: 1921
- AWPT Constitution and Bylaws: 1921
- American Physiotherapy Association (APA): 1922
- Minimum standard curriculum for schools: 1926
- Great Depression and Poliomyelitis
- Code of Ethics and Discipline
- National Foundation for Infantile Paralysis

History of the Physical Therapy Profession

Fundamental Accomplishment Years: 1940–1970

- Catherine Worthingham: President APA–1940–1945
- War Emergency Training Course of World War II: 1941–graduated Physiotherapy Aides
- United States Congress Bill–Physical Therapists: 1943
- APA's House of Delegates: 1944
- American Physical Therapy Association (APTA): 1946

History of the Physical Therapy Profession

Fundamental Accomplishment Years: 1940–1970
- Licensure laws: 1959
- PTs: clinical studies polio vaccine: 1948–1960
- Journal of Physical Therapy: 1964
- APTA–PTA creation: 1967
- Two PTA programs: 1969–Miami Dade CC in Miami; St. Mary's Campus of the College of St. Catherine in Minneapolis
- 15 PTA graduates: 1969

History of the Physical Therapy Profession

Mastery Years: 1970–1996
- Affiliate membership: 1970
- Commission on Accreditation in Physical Therapy Education (CAPTE): 1977
- Specialty sections: 1978
- American Board of Physical Therapy Specialties (ABPTS)
- Federation of State Boards of Physical Therapy (FSBPT): 1986
- Direct Access: 1988
- Affiliate Assembly: 1989
- 55% PT programs–Masters level: 1994
- 75 years of APTA: 1995

History of the Physical Therapy Profession

Adaptation and Vision Years: 1996 to present
- BBA: 1997 to present
- Normative Model of PTA Education: 1999
- PT Bulletin online: 2000
- Normative Model of PT Education: 2000
- *Guide to Physical Therapist Practice, Second Edition:* 2001
- Hooked on Evidence online: 2002
- Normative Model of PTA Education: 2006

History of the Physical Therapy Profession

Adaptation and Vision Years: 1996 to present
- Direct Access
- DPT programs
- PTA Caucus: 2005
- 66,037 APTA members: 2005
- APTA's 2020 Vision
- DPTs physical therapy providers
- PTAs assist DPTs
- PTAs: educated and licensed
- PTAs: physical therapist directed supervised components interventions

APTA's Benefits for Student Members

- ☐ Career guidance
- ☐ Member discounts
- ☐ Mentoring program
- ☐ Scholarship and internship
- ☐ Legislative representation
- ☐ E-newsletter

APTA's Goals

PTs
- Practitioners: choice, persons with conditions that affect movement and function
- Providers: fitness, health promotion, wellness,risk reduction programs, enhance quality of life persons across life span

PTs/PTAs
- Committed: meeting health needs patients/clients, society through ethical behavior, continued competence, collegial relationships other healthcare practitioners, advocacy profession

APTA Components
The House of Delegates

Components
- **52 chapters**
- **18 sections**
- **2 assemblies (PTA Caucus and Student Assembly)**

Annual meetings
- **CSM (February)**
- **Annual Conference and Exhibition (June)**

House of Delegates (HOD)
- **Highest policy making body of APTA**
- **Affiliate delegation (5 PTAs)**

APTA's Board of Directors
and Headquarters

- **Six officers**
- **President**
- **Vice President**
- **Secretary**
- **Treasurer**
- **Speaker of the House of Delegates**
- **Vice Speaker of the House of Delegates**
- **Headquarters: Alexandria, Virginia**
- **Online: www.apta.org**
- **Toll-free: 800-999-2782**

The Physical Therapist Assistant as a Member of the Healthcare Team

LEARNING OBJECTIVES

After studying Chapter 2, the reader will be able to:

- Discuss the supervisory role of the physical therapist on the health care team.
- Describe the differences in role, function, and supervisory relationships of the physical therapist, physical therapist assistant, and other health care personnel.
- Identify the use of the *Guide to Physical Therapist Practice.*
- List the events taking place in the collaborative path between physical therapist and physical therapist assistant.
- Compare and contrast the types of health care teams.
- Identify the members of the rehabilitation team and their responsibilities.
- Describe the five elements of patient and client management in physical therapy practice.
- List employment settings for physical therapists and physical therapist assistants.
- Compare and contrast the three types of skilled nursing facilities.
- Discuss employment and physical therapy clinical practice issues such as interviews, policy and procedure manuals, meetings, budgets, quality assurance, and risk management.

GLOSSARY

Assessment data: Data that include an appraisal or evaluation of a patient's condition based on clinical and laboratory data, medical history, and the patient's accounts of symptoms; data included in the "A" section of the SOAP note; in the SOAP note, they provide the rationale for the necessity of the skilled physical therapy services, interprets the data, and gives meaning to the data.

Disability: The inability to engage in age-specific, gender-related, and sex-specific roles in a particular social context and physical environment; it is also any restriction or lack (resulting from an injury) of ability to perform an activity in a manner or within the range considered normal for a human being.

Functional limitation: Restriction of the ability to perform a physical action, activity, or task in an efficient, typically expected, or competent manner.

Impairment: A loss or abnormality of psychological, physiological, or anatomical structure or function.

Medical diagnosis: Physician's identification of the cause of the patient's illness or discomfort.

Physical abuse: Abuse by grabbing, pinching, shoving, slapping, hitting, hair pulling, or biting; abuse by denying medical care or forcing alcohol and/or drug use.

Physical therapy diagnosis: The use of data obtained by physical therapy examination and other relevant information to determine the cause and nature of a patient's impairments, functional limitations, and disabilities.

Treatment plan: The projected series and sequence of treatment procedures based on an individualized evaluation of what is needed to restore or improve the health and function of a patient in physical therapy, the treatment plan gives direction to the medical care and provides an approach to measure the effectiveness of treatment.

Notes

CHAPTER 2

THE PHYSICAL THERAPIST ASSISTANT AS A MEMBER OF THE HEALTHCARE TEAM

THE GUIDE TO PHYSICAL THERAPIST PRACTICE

How To Use the Guide

- Framework for decision making
- Options for daily practice
- Terminology and thought processes
- Teaching tool
- Interpretation of clinical practice
- References
- Explanation/justification of interventions
- Research
- Legislature

Terminology Used in the Guide

- Patient: received physical therapy direct interventions
- Client: can benefit from PT's consultation
- Examination: gathers objective and subjective patient's/client's data
- Evaluation: PT's clinical judgments based on examination data
- Interventions: skilled techniques and activities in the treatment plan
- Discharge: discontinuing interventions in a single episode of care

Components of Physical Therapy Examination

- Patient/client history examples: past and current health status
- Systems review examples: cardiopulmonary, musculoskeletal
- Tests and measures: body mechanics, balance, MMT, ROM, pain, reflex integrity, motor function, orthotic devices

Evaluation Results

- Physical therapy diagnosis: different than medical diagnosis—established by MD/DO
- Impairments: dysfunctions of bones, joints, ligaments, tendons, muscles, nerves, skin, or movement pathology
- Functional limitations: inability to function example: inability to perform ADLs
- Disability: inability to perform at work, home, or community—example: inability to work
- Prognosis: PT's judgment of the patient's optimal level of improvement
- Physical therapy interventions

Physical Therapy Interventions and Discharge

- Interventions: PT/PTA purposeful and skilled interactions with patient/client, produce changes in the condition consistent with diagnosis and prognosis
- Interventions: coordination, communication, and documentation; patient/client related instruction; direct interventions
- Indications–discharge
- Patient's desire stop treatment
- Patient's inability to progress toward goals
- PT's decision patient will no longer benefit from physical therapy

Part Two of the Guide

- Contains prefer practice patterns: musculoskeletal, neuromuscular, cardiopulmonary, integumentary
- Practice patterns based: examination findings–impairments, functional limitations, disabilities
- Interventions-based disablement system: pathology, pathophysiology; impairments–functional limitations, disability

Notes

CHAPTER 2

THE PHYSICAL THERAPIST ASSISTANT AS A MEMBER OF THE HEALTHCARE TEAM

Definition and Supervision of PTA

- PTA: educated individual works under direction and supervision of PT
- Supervision of PTA: dependent clinical site jurisdiction
- PTA: graduate PTA program–CAPTE accredited
- General supervision: PT available telecommunication
- Direct personal supervision: PT available on-site at all times
- PT: conducts physical therapy practice

PTA Duties (as per the APTA)

- Performs selected physical therapy interventions under the direction and at least general supervision of PT–dependent on the jurisdiction of clinical site
- Makes modifications to selected interventions to progress the patient/client, as directed by the PT, or to ensure patient/client safety and comfort
- Documents patient's/client's progress
- Performs direct personal supervision—where allowable by law—of the physical therapy aide, PTA student, and other personnel

PT's Responsibilities while Supervising the PTA in Off-Site Setting

- ☐ PT accessible to PTA: telecommunications–dependent on jurisdiction clinical site
- ☐ Scheduled and documented conferences between PT and PTA: dependent on patient's/PTA's needs
- ☐ Supervisory visits by the PT
- Upon PTA's request patient's re-examination
- When POC change needed
- Prior planned discharge
- In response: change patient's medical status
- Once/month or higher frequency–patient's needs

Collaboration Path Between the PT and the PTA

1. PT performs initial examination/evaluation, establishes POC and treatment plan
2. PTA helps PT: initial examination/evaluation; PTA takes notes and gathers data as requested by PT
3. PT interprets the results of the data–called evaluation
4. PT performs patient's interventions–PTA performs selected patient's interventions as directed by PT

Collaboration Path Between the PT and the PTA

5. PTA performs data collection during interventions; PTA records patient's progress/lack of progress; PTA may ask PT for re-examination
6. PT performs re-examination and establishes new treatment plan
7. PT performs new patient's interventions–PTA performs new selected interventions as directed by PT
8. PT performs discharge examination and evaluation of patient

Types of Healthcare Teams

- Intradisciplinary: members work together within the same discipline–PT and PTA in home health care
- Interdisciplinary: members work together within all disciplines–SNF team: PT, PTA, SLP, OT, COTA, MD, RN, SW, LPN
- Multidisciplinary: members work separately and independently in different disciplines, different medical specialties–a patient with a specific pathology seen by different medical specialties to find a medical diagnosis

Rehabilitation Team

- PT and PTA
- OTR/L and COTA
- SLP
- Orthotist and Prosthetist
- Physician: Family and General Practitioner, Psychiatrist, Orthopedic Surgeon, Neurologist, Pediatrician
- RN, LPN, CNA
- SW
- ATC

Employment Settings for PTAs

- Acute care hospitals and rehabilitation hospitals
- Subacute care
- Subacute care SNF
- Transitional care SNF
- Extended care SNF
- Outpatient: orthopedic and sports, pediatric, women's health
- Home health care
- Hospice care
- School system
- Private practice

Physical Therapy Employment

- ☐ Interview preparation
- • Physical
- • Professional: starts in PTA program
- • Mental
- ☐ Resume
- • Chronological: used the most in health care
- • Functional
- ☐ References: dressing, communication skills
- ☐ Questions for prospective employer
- • Organization advantages/disadvantages
- • Benefits: working hours
- • Vacation: sick/personal leave time
- • Salary range: description job requirements

Policy and Procedure Manual and Departmental Meetings

- ☐ Policy and Procedure Manual
- • Policy: broad statement represents principle–law–decision–example: required and expected dress code
- • Procedure: sequence, steps required–performing policy action–examples: how to clean equipment, how to implement safety procedures
- ☐ Departmental meetings
- • Staff/departmental team: PT, PTA, OTR/L, COTA, SLP, SW, RN
- • Supervisory: PT and PTA
- • Strategic planning

Fiscal Management of Physical Therapy Service

- ☐ Budgets
- • Operating expense: salaries, benefits
- • Capital expense: equipment > $300
- • Accounts receivable: Medicare funds
- • Accounts payable: money for services or equipment
- ☐ Costs
- • Direct: salaries, equipment
- • Indirect: housekeeping, utilities
- • Variable: electricity
- • Fixed: rent

Quality Assurance

- ☐ **QA: monitors quality and appropriateness of care–resolves identified problems**
- ☐ **QA**
- **Utilization Review: evaluates necessity, effectiveness, efficiency**
- **Peer Review: evaluates and improves quality of work**
- **Risk Management: implements quality assurance and defends against legal liability threats (safety education, identify potential employee injuries, report all incidents)**

MAJOR PHYSICAL THERAPY PRACTICE SPECIALTIES

INTRODUCTION TO PART II

Part II of this textbook includes three chapters that describe the major physical therapy practice specialties. The chapters are:

- Chapter 3: Musculoskeletal (Orthopedic) Physical Therapy
- Chapter 4: Neurologic and Cardiopulmonary Physical Therapy
- Chapter 5: Pediatric, Geriatric, and Integumentary Physical Therapy

These three chapters classify physical therapy practices into six major divisions: musculoskeletal, neurologic, cardiopulmonary, pediatric, geriatric, and integumentary. Although physical therapists (PTs) can specialize in cardiovascular and pulmonary, clinical electrophysiologic, geriatric, neurologic, orthopedic, pediatric, and sports physical therapy, the clinical practices may include more than one of these specialties. For example, musculoskeletal (orthopedic) physical therapy clinical practices may contain physical therapy for rheumatologic conditions, orthopedic rehabilitation, sports injuries and treatments, manual therapy, low back pain, or aquatic physical therapy. Geriatric and pediatric patients can also be treated for musculoskeletal disorders in a musculoskeletal physical therapy practice.

However, as a specialty, musculoskeletal (orthopedic) physical therapy specializes in treating patients who have orthopedic disorders including sports injuries. Neurologic physical therapy specializes in treating patients who have neurologic disorders. Cardiopulmonary physical therapy specializes in treating patients who have cardiac and pulmonary conditions. Pediatric physical therapy specializes in treating children who have developmental dysfunction and specific pediatric disorders. Geriatric physical therapy specializes in treating older individuals who present with musculoskeletal and neuromuscular conditions and dysfunction common to the older adult. Integumentary physical therapy specializes in treating patients who have skin disorders including wounds and burns.

LABORATORY ACTIVITIES FOR PART II

The following activities are suggested to the instructor to involve students in the application of laboratory performances:

- Interview a PTA working in an orthopedic physical therapy clinical practice.
- Interview a PTA working in a neurologic physical therapy clinical practice.
- Interview a PTA working in a cardiopulmonary physical therapy clinical practice.
- Interview a PTA working in a pediatric physical therapy clinical practice.
- Interview a PTA working in a geriatric physical therapy clinical practice.
- Visit a wound care department, and then give a class presentation about wound physical therapy.

Musculoskeletal (Orthopedic) Physical Therapy

CHAPTER
3

LEARNING OBJECTIVES

After studying Chapter 3, the reader will be able to:

- Name the largest clinical specialty of physical therapy practice.
- Discuss the elements of a musculoskeletal examination. Compare and contrast examination, evaluation, and assessment.
- Identify the elements of patient history.
- Compare the two types of pain scales used frequently in physical therapy practice.
- Identify the basic activities of daily living and the instrumental activities of daily living.
- List the phases and subunits of the gait cycle.
- Identify the major orthopedic interventions and their roles in physical therapy practice.
- Discuss the types of therapeutic exercises used in musculoskeletal physical therapy including a home exercises program.
- Describe basic physical agents used in musculoskeletal physical therapy.
- Discuss patient education.
- Describe signs and symptoms and physical therapy interventions for degenerative osteoarthritis versus rheumatoid arthritis.
- Identify other musculoskeletal disorders (such as osteoporosis, tendonitis, bursitis, fractures, strains and sprains, and dislocations) and physical therapy interventions.
- Describe major types of orthopedic surgeries and physical therapy interventions.

GLOSSARY

Arthrography: A contrast medium such as iodine is injected into the joint and X-rays are taken to create images of the contours of the joint.

Capsular pattern: Pattern of limitation and restriction at the joint due to tightness or rigidity of the joint capsule.

Cryotherapy: Therapeutic application of cold such as ice or cold pack.

Computed Tomography (CT) scan: A scanning procedure that produces a type of X-ray image in a cross-sectional view; used to scan internal body structures.

Contralateral: Affecting the opposite side of the injury.

Electrotherapy: The use of electrical stimulation modalities in physical therapy treatment.

Hydrotherapy: Physical therapy intervention using water.

Hypertrophy: Increased cell size leading to increases in tissue size.

Hypomobility: Condition of restricted motion in a joint; decreasing mobility of the joint.

Ischemia: Reduced oxygen supply to a body organ or part; lack of blood supply to a body organ or part due to functional constriction or actual obstruction of a blood vessel.

Proprioceptive neuromuscular facilitation (PNF): A form of therapeutic exercise in which accommodating resistance is manually applied to various patterns of movement for the purpose of strengthening the muscles.

Magnetic resonance imaging (MRI): A scanning technique using magnetic fields and radio frequencies to produce a precise image of the body tissue; the images have very good anatomic detail.

Microtrauma: Very small injury.

Noncapsular pattern: Pattern of limitations and restrictions at the joint indicating fragments of bone or tissue floating around the joint.

Orthopedic shoes: Shoes specially made for sensitive deformed structures of the foot that distribute the weight toward a pain-free area.

Orthosis: A device added to a person's body to support, position, or immobilize a part to correct deformities; to assist weak muscles; and restore function.

Parenteral: Any medication route other than the alimentary canal, such as intravenous, subcutaneous, intramuscular, or mucosal.

Pronation: The act of assuming the prone position; turning or rotation of the hand so that the palm is facing down towards the floor.

Resorbed: Absorbed.

Slow stroking: A neurological technique consisting of continuous slow stroking to spinal posterior primary rami to produce a calming effect and generalized inhibition.

Subchondral: Below or under a cartilage.

Subluxation: Partial or incomplete dislocation of the joint.

Thermotherapy: Intervention through the application of heat.

Vasodilation: Increase in the diameter of blood vessels, which increases blood flow.

Notes

CHAPTER 3

MUSCULOSKELETAL (ORTHOPEDIC) PHYSICAL THERAPY

Physical Therapy Goals in Musculoskeletal Clinical Practice

- Maximize patient's function
- Alleviate patient's pain
- Decrease abnormal joint stress
- Patient's utilization of proper posture
- Promote tissue healing, range of motion, and flexibility

Patient History

- Age, gender, occupation
- Medical diagnosis and physical therapy precautions
- Patient's chief complaint (reason for assistance)
- Present illness (symptoms, location, severity)
- Mechanism of injury (trauma), symptoms progression
- Past history (X-rays, prior treatments, general health)
- Patient's lifestyle (occupation, sports, family)

Pain Description

- Taken prior and after treatment
- Elements: location, radiation, intensity, duration, frequency, progression, aggravating and relieving factors, prior test results for pain
- Pain measurements

Visual Analog Scale (VAS): 10cm unmarked vertical/horizontal line

Numerical Rating System (NRS): easier to use; uses a number such as 0–10

Examples of Musculoskeletal Assessments

- Posture
- ROM: PROM and AROM—goniometer
- MMT: normal, good, fair, poor, trace, absent
- ADLs: BADLs (dressing, bathing) and IADLs (shopping, driving)
- DTRs: C5-biceps brachii; L3-quadriceps
- Gait
- Traditional (older): stance (60% gait cycle) and swing (40% gait cycle)
- RLA (newer)

Musculoskeletal Interventions

Therapeutic exercises
- ROM: AROM–increase strength; PROM–does not increase strength; AAROM–increase strength–manual/mechanical assistance
- Strengthening: isometric–no joint motion; CKC– functional; OKC–non weight bearing postures; isotonic–manual/mechanical resistance, PREs, PNFs; isokinetic–specialized machines
- Stretching: manual passive, self, ballistic
- Relaxation

Musculoskeletal Interventions

- ❑ **Physical Agents and Modalities**
- • Thermotherapy–superficial heating agents—MHP, paraffin; deep heating agents–ultrasound, diathermy
- • Cryotherapy–cold packs, ice cubes for ice massage, vapocoolant spray, contrast baths
- • Hydrotherapy–whirlpool, Hubbard tank–low boy; aquatic therapy–pool
- • Electrotherapy–NMES–strengthening; HVPC–edema; Iontophoresis–pain and inflammation; TENS–pain management; EMG Biofeedback–strengthening and relaxation; IFC–pain relief

Musculoskeletal Interventions

- ❑ **Therapeutic massage**
- • Effleurage
- • Petrissage
- • Friction
- • Percussion
- • Vibration
- ❑ **Manipulation and mobilization**
- ❑ **Mechanical spinal traction**
- • Cervical
- • Lumbar
- ❑ **Gait training**
- ❑ **Orthotics and prosthetics**

Musculoskeletal Disorders and Interventions

DJD: decrease pain and inflammation; promote function with modifications; decrease weakness and increase flexibility

RA: modalities and exercises to prevent deformities and maintain ROM

Osteoporosis: restore mobility, function, strength, confidence

Tendonitis: reduction of pain (RICE, massage), correct muscle imbalances, restore function

Bursitis: rest the area (RICE), bracing, promote function

Musculoskeletal Disorders and Interventions

Sprain–ligament tear

Strain–muscle/tendon tear

- **Sprain grade 3–may require surgery**
- **Sprain/strain–no surgery interventions: RICE, maintain ROM, decrease pain, stretching, functional strengthening, patient education**

Fractures

- **During immobilization–strengthen uninvolved extremity and body conditioning**
- **After surgery–PROM and AROM exercises, later PREs**

Post Surgery Orthopedic Physical Therapy Interventions

THR

- **Patient education for hip precautions, bed mobility, transfers and gait training with weight bearing restrictions, isometric exercises, return to function**

ACL Reconstruction

- **Bracing, isometric exercises, patellar mobs, modalities for swelling, OKC, CKC, and proprioceptive and balance exercises**

Discectomies

- **Patient education for back protection (no bending, lifting, twisting), return to function**

Neurologic and Cardiopulmonary Physical Therapy

LEARNING OBJECTIVES

After studying Chapter 4, the reader will be able to:

- List Kubler-Ross' five stages of adjustment to disease or loss.
- List specific elements of the neurologic examination.
- Describe specific neurologic physical therapy treatments to improve motor control and motor learning.
- Identify the major neurologic disorders (such as stroke, traumatic brain injury, or Parkinson's disease) and related physical therapy treatments.
- Describe the specific physical therapy examination and evaluation elements used by the physical therapist (PT) in cardiopulmonary physical therapy practice.
- Name specific interventions used in cardiopulmonary physical therapy.
- Discuss the major cardiopulmonary diseases (such as coronary artery disease or chronic obstructive pulmonary disease) and related physical therapy interventions.

GLOSSARY

Angina pectoris: Substernal chest pain or pressure due to insufficient flow of blood to the heart muscle.

Aphasia: Neurological impairment of language comprehension, formulation, and use; patients have deficits in speech, writing, or sign communication.

Apraxia: The inability to initiate and perform voluntary purposeful movements.

Approximation: Neurological intervention using compression forces applied to joints by gravity acting on the body weight.

Atherosclerosis: Fatty or cholesterol-lipid-calcium deposited in the walls of arteries, veins, and the lymphatic system.

"

Atherosclerotic: Caused by atherosclerosis.

Barrel chest: An increased anteroposterior chest diameter caused by increased functional residual capacity due to loss of elastic recoil in the lung.

Bradykinesia: Slowness of body movement and speech; can be found in Parkinson's disease.

Cardiac decompensation: Failure of the heart to maintain adequate circulation; failure of other organs to work properly.

Cerebral embolism: The obstruction of a blood vessel by an embolus in the brain.

Cerebral hemorrhage: Abnormal bleeding as a result of rupture of a blood vessel.

Congestive heart failure: The inability of the heart to pump enough blood to maintain adequate circulation of the blood to meet the body's metabolic needs.

Dementia: A progressive, irreversible decline in mental function.

Demyelination: Destruction or removal of the myelin sheath of nerve tissue.

Denervated muscles: Muscles in which the afferent and efferent nerves are cut.

Dyspnea: Inability or difficulty breathing (shortness of breath).

Dystonia: Impaired tone due to prolonged muscular contractions causing twisting of body parts.

Edema: Accumulation of large amounts of fluid in the tissues of the body; swelling.

Egophony: Abnormal change in tone of voice; sounds like a bleat of a goat; patients with pleural effusions or pneumonia sound egophony during auscultation of the chest.

Embolus: A mass of undissolved matter present in a blood or lymphatic vessel and brought there by the blood or lymph; can produce occlusion in the arteries, veins, or lymph system.

Encephalitis: Inflammation of the white and gray matter of the brain; can be caused by viruses, rabies, flu, acquired immune deficiency syndrome (AIDS), or fungi.

Flaccidity: A state of low tone in the muscle that produces weak and floppy limbs.

Hemiparesis: Weakness of the left or right side of the body.

Hemiplegia: Condition in which half of the body is paralyzed; paralysis.

Homonymous hemianopsia: Blindness of the nasal half of the visual field of one eye and temporal half of the visual field of the other eye.

Hypertonia: Increased tone above normal resting level.

Hypotonia: Decreased tone below normal resting level.

Idiopathic: Designating a disease whose cause is unknown.

Impairment: A loss or abnormality of psychological, physiological, or anatomical structure or function.

Kinesthetic sense: The ability to sense the direction of movement.

Myocardial infarction (MI): Heart attack resulting from obstruction of blood circulation to an area of the heart.

Paranoia: A condition in which patients show persistent persecutory delusions or delusional jealousy; in patients who are middle age or older, paranoia can also manifest with resentment, anger, and violence.

Pectoriloquy: The vocal sounds seem to emanate from the patient's chest (upon auscultation with a stethoscope); patient may have a pleural effusion.

Plasmapheresis: The removal of plasma from a patient to treat an illness and replacement with normal plasma.

Postencephalitic: Occurring after encephalitis; an abnormal state remaining after the acute stage of encephalitis.

Proprioception: The awareness of posture, movement, and changes in equilibrium and the knowledge of position, weight, and resistance of objects in relation to the body; proprioception includes awareness of the joints at rest and with movement.

Proprioceptive neuromuscular facilitation (PNF): A form of therapeutic exercise in which accommodating resistance is manually applied to various patterns of movement for the purpose of strengthening the muscles.

Resting tremor: Tremor present when the involved part is at rest but absent or diminished when active movement is attempted; can be found in Parkinson's disease.

Rigidity: Hypertonicity of muscles offering a constant, uniform resistance to passive movement; the affected muscles are unable to relax and in a state of contraction even at rest.

Rhythmic initiation: A neurological facilitation technique of PNF; therapeutic exercise performed in physical therapy using a voluntary relaxation followed by passive movements, then active assisted movements progressing to resisted movements; it may be used in Parkinson's disease to facilitate movement.

Spasticity: Increase in muscle tone and stretch reflex of a muscle resulting in increased resistance to passive stretch of the muscle and high response to sensory stimulation.

Thrombosis: Coagulation of the blood in the heart or a blood vessel forming a clot or a thrombus.

Tracheostomy: The surgical opening of the trachea to provide an open airway.

Ventilation: The movement of air into and out of the lungs.

Notes

CHAPTER 4

NEUROLOGICAL AND CARDIOPULMONARY PHYSICAL THERAPY

Psychosocial Stages of Adjustment in Neurological Rehab

- Denial: after discovering the disease/loss
- Anger: blame and hostility
- Bargaining: negotiations to change the situation
- Depression: loss of interest in living
- Acceptance: coming to terms with the disease/loss

Examples of Neurological Assessments

- Cranial nerve examination
- Muscle tone assessment
- Posture assessment
- Balance and coordination assessments
- Attention–environmental awareness; orientation–awareness to time, person, place; cognition assessments–memory, judgment, language
- Hearing and vision assessments
- Sensory assessments: pain, temperature, light touch, kinesthesia, proprioception

Neurophysiological Approaches

- **Neurodevelopmental treatment (NDT)–Karl and Berta Bobath–promotes normal movement sequence; inhibits abnormal tone**
- **Proprioceptive neuromuscular facilitation (PNF)–Kabat, Knott, Voss–spiral and diagonal patterns for function**
- **Sensory stimulation techniques–Rood– facilitation and inhibition techniques**
- **Movement therapy–Brunnstrom–used in hemiplegia–relearn the movement**

Examples of Neurological Disorders and Interventions

- ☐ **Acute CVA**
- **Positioning supine, sidelying, prone, sitting**
- **Skin integrity**
- **No traction injuries to affected arm Facilitation techniques: tapping vibration**
- **Weight bearing position–involved extremity**
- **Rolling onto affected side with sidelying position; sidelying on elbow position**
- **Supine to sit transfers, sitting, bridging**
- **Standing, walking, lateral/rotational weight shifts**
- **Scooting in sitting–ensures mobility dressing**

Examples of Neurological Disorders and Interventions

- ☐ **TBI–Rancho LOCF I, II, III**
- **ROM, prevent contracture: PROM, positioning, splinting, serial casting**
- **Skin integrity**
- **Respiratory status: postural drainage, percussion, vibration**
- **Sensory stimulation for arousal and to elicit movement–use auditory, visual, olfactory, gustatory, tactile stimuli**
- **Functional mobility skills–upright positioning and proper body alignment**

Examples of Neurological Disorders and Interventions

- PD: AROM, strength, gait, flexibility, balance, posture, ADLs, diaphragmatic breathing
- C6 SCI: bed mobility with rails; weight shifting–pressure relief; powered wheelchair training; manual wheelchair training; sliding board transfers
- Bell's Palsy: facial strengthening exercises–use ES; eye patch
- Alzheimer's disease: safety–monitoring devices; prevent falls; safe walking program; balance activities; family education
- Guillain-Barre syndrome: PROM, gait training, balance, ADLs, strengthening exercises, home/community integration

Examples of Cardiopulmonary Assessments

- Temperature
- Vital Signs: BP, Pulse, Respiration
- Auscultation: breath sounds–crackles, wheezes
- Skin color: cyanotic skin–nail beds
- Edema
- Current medications: alter vital signs
- Cough: sputum production–color, viscosity, amount
- Exercise Tolerance Test–PT evaluates patient; PTA may perform

Examples of Cardiopulmonary Interventions

- Cardiac Rehab: Phase I–hospital; Phase II–outpatient; Phase III–community outpatient
- Postural drainage: sitting, semi-reclined, supine, prone, sidelying, Trendelenburg
- Percussion: rhythmic force patient's chest wall–cupping
- Vibration: bouncing technique in inhalation and exhalation
- Coughing techniques: example–huffing–inhale deep–expel air saying "ha, ha"

Examples of Cardiopulmonary Diseases and Interventions

- ❑ CAD: patient education vital signs prior, during, after exercises/activities; cardiac rehab stages
- ❑ COPD: vital signs; patient/family education deep coughing; deep breathing exercises; postural/shoulders ROM exercises
- ❑ Asthma: pursed lip/diaphragmatic breathing; relaxation exercises
- ❑ Pneumonia: postural drainage, percussion, vibration, diaphragmatic breathing, coughing techniques

Pediatric, Geriatric, and Integumentary Physical Therapy

LEARNING OBJECTIVES

After studying Chapter 5, the reader will be able to:

- List the specific physical therapy examination and evaluation elements used by the physical therapist in pediatric physical therapy practice.
- Describe specific interventions common in pediatric physical therapy.
- Discuss the major pediatric diseases (such as cerebral palsy, Down's syndrome, or Duchenne muscular dystrophy) and related physical therapy interventions.
- Name specific elements used by the physical therapist in the initial examination and evaluation of the geriatric patient.
- List specific age-related changes of the older adult significant when providing physical therapy interventions.
- Describe specific geriatric diseases and limitations (such as immobility or fractures) and related physical therapy treatments.
- List elements of wound and burn assessment.
- Describe major physical therapy interventions for wound and burn care.

GLOSSARY

Apgar score: A system of evaluating an infant's physical condition at birth, discovered by Virginia Apgar, an American anesthesiologist; the infant's heart rate, respiration, muscle tone, response to stimuli, and color are rated at 1 minute, and again at 5 minutes after birth.

Asphyxia: Condition of insufficient intake of oxygen.

Cerebral hemorrhage: Abnormal bleeding as a result of rupture of a blood vessel.

Hydrotherapy: Physical therapy intervention using water.

Hypertonia: Increased tone above normal resting level.

Impairment: A loss or abnormality of psychological, physiological, or anatomical structure or function.

Perinatal: Time period immediately before and after birth.

Spasticity: Increase in muscle tone and stretch reflex of a muscle resulting in increased resistance to passive stretch of the muscle and high response to sensory stimulation.

Notes

CHAPTER 5

**PEDIATRIC, GERIATRIC, AND
INTEGUMENTARY PHYSICAL
THERAPY**

Pediatric Team

- PT: direct care provider–Early Intervention Programs (EIPs)
- PTA: under PT direct supervision–dependent jurisdiction
- Patient and Patient family
- MD/DO
- RN
- OTR/L and COTA
- SLP and Psychologist
- Teachers and Special educators

Examples of Pediatric Assessments

- Neonatal reflexes
- Babinski: 0–12 months–stroking lateral aspect of plantar surface of foot = toes extension/fanning
- Symmetrical Tonic Neck Reflex (STNR): 6–8 months–neck flexion = arms in flexion and legs in extension; neck extension = arms in extension and legs in flexion
- Developmental Milestones by Age: assess gross and fine motor functions, language, social, adaptive skills (such coordination), and cognitive skills–from birth to adolescence (13–18 years)

Examples of Pediatric Interventions

- Orthopedic: bracing, PROM/AROM exercises, stretching, strengthening, mobility training (rolling walker), orthotics, balance/endurance, compensatory techniques
- Neurological: positioning, neurophysiological approaches, adaptive equipment (prone stander), ROM, mobility training, exercises, family education, functional skills
- Pulmonary: percussion, postural drainage, aerobic activity (loosen secretions)
- Developmental disability: orthosis, mobility training, adaptive equipment

Examples of Pediatric Disorders and Interventions

- CP: individualized interventions–team approach – example: hypertonia CP– positioning hips and knees > 90 degrees of flexion, inhibition of abnormal reflexes, weight bearing activities
- Down Syndrome: facilitate lip closure, inhibit tongue protrusion, positioning, strengthening, education C1–C2 vertebral instability
- Duchenne Muscular Dystrophy: stretching, ambulation assistive devices, braces, ADLs, recreation (pool therapy)

Examples of Pediatric Disorders and Interventions

- Scoliosis: bracing (Milwaukee orthosis), stretching tight muscles (concave), strengthen weak muscles (convex)
- Spina Bifida
- Family education
- Positioning: minimize deformity
- Strengthening: playing
- Stretching
- Static/dynamic stander: positioning upright
- Orthotic devices

Focus of Geriatric Rehab

- Patient/client: unique
- Functional goals
- Optimal health
- Highest level of function
- Patient's decision making: autonomy
- Cultural and ethnic sensitivity
- Comfort and coping skills
- Consider whole patient: holism
- Effective communication
- Advocate for needed services

Examples of Geriatric Assessments

- Physical assessment: dependent on pathology (such as orthopedic)
- Functional assessment:
  - Mobility, hobbies, social
  - Sensory function: vision, hearing, balance
  - Motor function: strength, endurance, gait, skeletal changes, risk of falls
  - Mental function: memory, learning
- Psychosocial assessment: Mental Status Questionnaire; Geriatric Depression Scale
- Environmental assessment: home, institution

Clinical Considerations During Geriatric Interventions

- Slower movement and increased fatigue
- Risk of muscle/ligament tear
- Increased adhesions
- Decreased speed in ambulation, shorter steps, less arm swing
- Increased reliance on vision for movement
- Visual and hearing deficits
- Sensory losses: touch, taste, smell
- Various strategies for memory and learning
- Cardiac output at rest—unchanged
- Breathing difficulties with exercises
- Effects of medications, nutrition, family

Notes

Examples of Integumentary Assessments

Skin assessments
- ☐ Lesion characteristics—ex: elevated
- ☐ Edema or swelling; nail condition
- ☐ Skin temperature, color, and pigmentation
- ☐ Pain, increased perspiration, unusual growths

Wound assessments
- ☐ Location and measurement—edges, depth
- ☐ Size, drainage, and granulation
- ☐ Edema and skin changes

Burn assessments: classification of burn area, degree, complications, healing, management

Examples of Integumentary Interventions

- ☐ Skin disorders/dysfunctions
- Patient education; Exercises; ADLs
- Skin protection; Modalities: ultrasound, ultraviolet, aquatic, paraffin, fluidotherapy
- ☐ Wounds
- Cleansing: whirlpool, pulsatile lavage
- Modalities: as per PT treatment plan
- Debridement; Dressing: as per MD/DO
- ☐ Burns
- Debridement and positioning
- ROM exercises, pressure garments, breathing exercises, infection control

ETHICAL AND LEGAL ISSUES

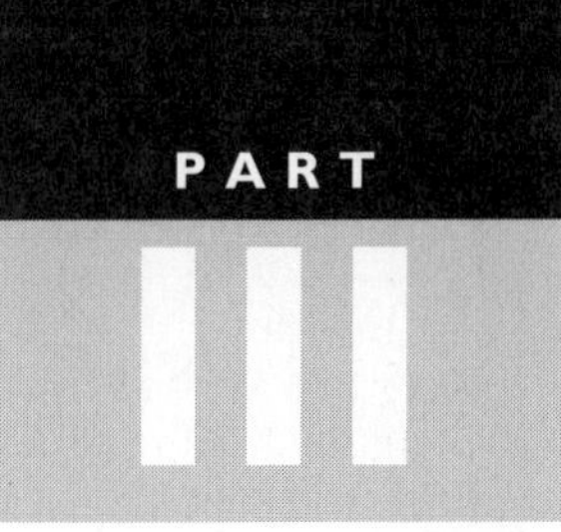

INTRODUCTION TO PART III

Part III of the text describes ethical issues encountered in physical therapy, including professionalism and laws and regulations pertaining to the physical therapist and physical therapist assistant. Part III contains two chapters:

- Chapter 6: Ethics and Professionalism
- Chapter 7: Law and Regulations

LABORATORY ACTIVITIES FOR PART III

The following activities are suggested to the instructor to involve students in the application of laboratory performances:

- Read the APTA's guide for professional conduct for PTs, and identify at least four directive ethical principles that, if broken, can also constitute a violation of the law.
- Read the APTA's guide for conduct for PTAs and identify at least four directive ethical principles that, if broken, can also constitute a violation of the law.
- Give at least two examples of the beneficence principle that can apply to physical therapy.
- Give at least two examples of the nonmaleficence principle that can apply to physical therapy.
- Interview a PTA about standards of cultural and linguistic competence in his or her clinical settings.
- Give a class presentation about patient confidentiality in physical therapy practice including HIPAA's standards in regard to reasonable safeguards that a physical therapy provider must implement.
- Give a class presentation about a patient's informed consent in physical therapy practice.
- Perform an accessibility audit at your school to identify barriers and obstacles faced by students or faculty with disabilities.
- Interview a PTA working in a pediatric setting or a school about the IDEA and physical therapy interventions.
- Perform an Internet search about your state's licensure statutes determining physical therapy practice criteria.
- Perform an Internet search about the OSHA's news in regard to health care.
- Perform an Internet search about OSHA's blood-borne pathogens standard (BPS).
- Write a paper about domestic violence issues in your state and the applicable laws.
- Write a case scenario about a PTA who caused harm to a patient, being liable for negligence.

Ethics and Professionalism

After studying Chapter 6, the reader will be able to:

- Define morals and ethics.
- Delineate the difference between medical law and medical ethics.
- List six biomedical ethical principles and their roles in health care.
- Discuss patient confidentiality.
- Describe the Health Insurance Portability and Accountability Act (HIPAA) of 1996.
- Discuss the patient's bill of rights and its importance to physical therapy practice.
- Explain cultural competence in health care and physical therapy.
- List the elements of full informed consent.
- Explain the guide for professional conduct that physical therapists are morally bound to follow.
- Explain the guide for conduct of the affiliate member that physical therapist assistants are morally bound to follow.
- Identify at least five directive ethical provisions expected of the physical therapist assistant.

GLOSSARY

Emotional abuse: Undermining a person's sense of self-worth such as criticizing constantly, calling names, belittling one's abilities, or damaging a partner's relationship with the children.

Ethnocentrism: The universal tendency of human beings to think that their ways of thinking, acting, and believing are the only right, proper, and natural ways; universal phenomena in that most people tend to believe that their ways of living, believing, and acting are right, proper, and morally correct.

Notes

CHAPTER 6

ETHICS AND PROFESSIONALISM

Physical Therapy Ethics

- ❑ Physical therapy ethics: professional/moral standards PTs/PTAs
  - APTA Code of Ethics
  - APTA Guide for Professional Conduct
  - APTA Standards of Ethical Conduct
  - APTA Guide for Conduct of the Affiliate Member
- ❑ Physical therapy ethics violation: APTA's *Disciplinary Action Procedural Document*– investigation and hearing of claims
- ❑ Physical therapy laws violation: criminal and civil liability

---

Biomedical Ethical Principles

- ❑ Beneficence: act in patients' interest
- ❑ Nonmaleficence: do not cause harm to patient
- ❑ Justice: apply fair and equal treatment
- ❑ Veracity: provide truthful information
- ❑ Confidentiality: do not share or divulge patient information
- ❑ Autonomy: respect patients' rights

<hr>

Confidentiality

- ☐ PTA refers to supervising PT: all requests release confidential information
- ☐ Patient's information not confidential
- · Rare instances
- · Threat to patient/health of public
- · Federal Statutes
- ☐ Patient's written authorization for release of medical information needed
- · Insurance and attorney
- · Employer: except workers compensation
- · Family: except member–power of attorney

<hr>

Confidentiality

- ☐ HIPAA 1996: federal law
- ☐ Privacy Rule–CE: health plans–providers–clearinghouses
- · Notify patients privacy rights: first date of service– patient's written acknowledgment
- · Implement procedures
- · Train employees and secure records
- · Designate privacy officer
- ☐ PHI health information: any form or media
- ☐ Safeguards PHI
- · Speak quietly patient's condition
- · Do not use patient's name in public
- · Lock patient's records use computer passwords

<hr>

Confidentiality

- ☐ Patient authorization not needed for PHI
- · Patient's own PHI
- · DHHS
- · Required by law
- · Federal and state
- · Domestic/elder abuse
- · Workers compensation
- · Emergency situations
- ☐ PTA students
- · Patient authorization
- · Deidentify patient information before sharing

Confidentiality

- ☐ Patient entitled receive from CE
- • PHI during six years prior to request date
- • Name entity received/used PHI
- • Brief description PHI
- • Brief statement: purpose of disclosure
- ☐ CE can not use PHI marketing
- ☐ Violation of HIPAA–complaint driven
- • Civil penalties–fines
- • Criminal sanctions

Elements of Informed Consent

- ☐ Clear description of intervention–layperson's terms
- ☐ Reasonable alternatives proposed intervention
- ☐ Risks or benefits: uncertainties–each intervention
- ☐ Assessment patient's understanding
- ☐ Patient's acceptance intervention
- ☐ Patient competent
- ☐ Patient's consent voluntary
- ☐ Legal guardian's consent: minor or adult who is not competent

Role of Cultural Diversity

- ☐ Awareness/understanding/acceptance–Patient
- • Racial characteristics
- • National origin
- • Religious affiliations
- • Physical size–spoken language
- • Age–gender
- • Sexual orientation
- • Physical/mental disability
- • Socioeconomic/occupational status
- • Political orientation–geographical location

Cultural Competence

Ethical perspective
- ☐ Evolving process
- ☐ Acceptance/respect differences
- ☐ Self-assessment
- ☐ Expansion cultural knowledge/resources
- ☐ Vigilance toward dynamics of differences
- ☐ Adaptation to services

Legal perspective
- ☐ Federal standards
- ☐ JCAHO
- ☐ National Committee for Quality Assurance
- ☐ CAPTE

Develop Cultural Competence in Physical Therapy

- ☐ Identify personal cultural biases
- ☐ Understand cultural differences–seek knowledge about different cultures
- ☐ Diversity: acknowledge, accept, appreciate, value, and respond; do not avoid, minimize, tolerate, or be afraid
- ☐ Apply cultural competence clinical practice
- ☐ Developing cultural competence
- · An ongoing learning process
- · A slow process
- · Not an unmistakable process

Laws and Regulations

LEARNING OBJECTIVES

After studying Chapter 7, the reader will be able to:

- Identify the four primary sources of law in the United States.
- Describe the American with Disabilities Act of 1990.
- List the main points of Title I of the Americans with Disabilities Act and its effect on businesses and employers.
- Discuss the Individuals with Disabilities Education Act of 1997.
- Describe the role of licensure laws.
- List the name of the organization responsible for creating and managing the National Physical Therapy Examination for physical therapists and physical therapist assistants.
- Explain four minimum standards to enter the profession for physical therapists and physical therapist assistants.
- Describe the Occupational Safety and Health Administration and its role in health care.
- Discuss the importance of the blood-borne pathogens standard in health care, including physical therapy practice.
- Identify the Violence Against Women Act of 2000 and domestic violence issues in the United States.
- Describe domestic violence responses in health care and physical therapy.
- Identify two types of malpractice laws that can affect physical therapist assistants.

GLOSSARY

Blood-borne pathogens: Pathogenic microorganisms that are present in human blood and that can infect and cause disease in persons who are exposed to blood containing these pathogens; examples of blood-borne pathogens are hepatitis B and HIV.

Disability: The inability to engage in age-specific, gender-related, and sex-specific roles in a particular social context and physical environment; it is also any restriction or lack (resulting from an injury) of ability to perform an activity in a manner or within the range considered normal for a human being.

Domestic violence: A pattern of abusive behavior, which keeps one partner in a position of power over the other partner through the use of fear, intimidation, and control.

Economic abuse: Attempting or making a person financially dependent such as maintaining total control over financial resources, withholding access money, or forbidding attendance at school or employment.

Emotional abuse: Undermining a person's sense of self-worth such as criticizing constantly, calling names, belittling one's abilities, or damaging a partner's relationship with the children.

Exposure incident: A specific exposure to the eye, mouth, other mucous membrane; nonintact skin; or parenteral exposure to blood or other potentially infectious materials that results from the performance of an employee's duties.

Psychological abuse: Abuse causing fear by intimidation; threatening physical harm to self, partner, or children; destruction of pets and property; mind games or forcing isolation from friends, family, school and/or work.

Sexual abuse: Abuse by coercing or attempting to coerce any sexual contact without consent, abuse by marital rape, forcing sex after physical beating, attacks on sexual parts of the body, or treating another in a sexually demeaning manner.

Notes

CHAPTER 7

LAW AND REGULATIONS

Sources of Laws

- Constitutional: Federal Constitution laws–Bill of Rights; State constitutional laws–subordinated to federal
- Statutory: created by federal/state legislatures–Medicare, Medicaid, ADA
- Common: created by judges–malpractice laws
- Administrative–regulatory: created by federal, state, and local administrative agencies like OSHA

Americans with Disabilities Act (ADA)

- ADA–5 titles: prevents discrimination against persons with disabilities in certain areas
  - Employment
  - Public accommodation
  - State/local government services
  - Telecommunication
- Disability
  - Physical/mental impairment
  - Person has record of such impairment
  - Person regarded having such impairment

Americans with Disabilities Act (ADA)

- ☐ Reasonable accommodations: changes to work environment–permit employee or applicant to:
- Participate in job application process
- Perform essential functions of job
- Enjoy equal benefits and privileges of employment
- ☐ Employer: changing accommodation–undue hardship
- Disruptive and very costly
- Difficult to implement
- Fundamentally alters nature business

Individuals with Disabilities Education Act (IDEA)

- ☐ Purposes
- Free public education: special education and related services–children with disabilities from 3–21 years
- Protected rights: children with disabilities and parents
- Early intervention services infants and toddlers with disabilities from birth to 2 years
- Necessary tools: educators/parents
- Assess/ensure IDEA effectiveness

Individuals with Disabilities Education Act (IDEA)

- ☐ Related services
- Physical and Occupational therapy
- Audiology and Psychological services
- Transportation and Speech pathology
- Recreation, Counseling and Medical service
- ☐ Physical therapy services: promotion of sensorimotor function to enhance:
- Musculoskeletal/cardiopulmonary status
- Neurobehavioral organization
- Perceptual and motor development
- Environmental adaptation

Licensure Laws

- ❑ **Licensure laws**
- **Right to practice profession**
- **Protect consumer**
- **Regulatory practice acts**
- ❑ **Minimum standards PT/PTA licensure**
- **Graduation accredited PT/PTA programs**
- **Passed NPTE (minimum score 600)**
- **Knowledge ethical/legal standards**
- **PT/PTA license**

Occupational Safety and Health Administration (OSHA)

- ❑ **Mission**
- **Safety and Health American workers**
- **Training: outreach and education**
- **Partnerships**
- **Improvement workplace safety and health**
- ❑ **Bloodborne Pathogens Standard (BPS):**
- **Employee education/follow up: HBV/HIV– bloodborne diseases/prevention– communicable diseases**
- **Use safe/adequate protective equipment**
- **HBV vaccine**
- **Disposal: waste/sharp items**

Occupational Safety and Health Administration (OSHA)

- ❑ **PTs/PTAs–category 2: ECP**
- ❑ **Maintenance training records: 3 years**
- ❑ **Infection control**
- **Universal precautions**
- **Engineering controls**
- **Work practice controls**
- ❑ **Universal precautions**
- **Protective equipment**
- **Proper containers: waste**
- **Clean: work/patient area**
- **Hand washing**
- **Exposure report**

Domestic Violence

- ❑ **National Hotline: 800-799-7233**
- ❑ **Domestic violence**
- • **Coercion and threats**
- • **Intimidation and isolation**
- • **Emotional, sexual, or physical abuse**
- ❑ **Abuser methods**
- • **Sexual violence: uses children as pawns**
- • **Denies abuse, blames partner, controls finances, hurts children/pets**
- • **Instills fear, destroys property, insults, criticizes—partner is servant**
- • **Partner cannot leave house**

Domestic Violence in Physical Therapy

- ❑ **Victim's signs**
- • **Abuser accompanies victim, cancels appointments, visits multiple therapists**
- • **Victim missing appointments**
- • **Victim not allowed medications, victim lacks transportation and finances**
- ❑ **Victim screening**
- • **Chronic pain/injuries, injuries while pregnant**
- • **Poorly controlled chronic illnesses**
- • **Gynecological problems, anxiety, depression, easily startled**
- • **Suicide attempts, eating disorders, self mutilation, overuse pain medications**

Malpractice Laws

- ❑ **Negligence**
- • **Failure to give reasonable care**
- • **Failure to perform "a duty of care"**
- • **Harm occurred to patient**
- • **Patient suffered legally cognizable damages**
- ❑ **Malpractice acts physical therapy**
- • **Burns: defective equipment–ultrasound burn**
- • **Use defective equipment–wheelchair**
- • **Falls**
- • **Exercise injuries**
- • **Action/inaction inconsistent APTA's ethics**

COMMUNICATION

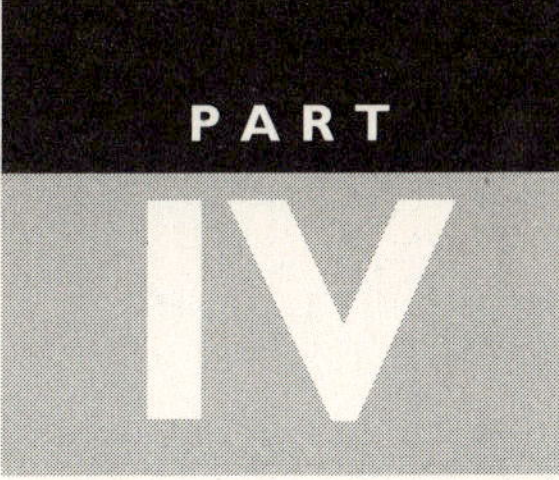

Part IV of this text discusses communication in health care and physical therapy and is divided into four chapters. These chapters are:

- Chapter 8: Communication Basics
- Chapter 9: Documentation and the Medical Record
- Chapter 10: Teaching, Learning, and Medical Terminology
- Chapter 11: Reimbursement and Research

LABORATORY ACTIVITIES FOR PART IV

The following activities are suggested to the instructor to involve students in the application of laboratory performances:

- Perform a role-play situation using correct verbal communication while trying to establish a rapport with the patient.
- Adapt verbal communication to reflect sensitivity to cultural differences in a role-play situation while trying to establish a rapport with the patient.
- Engage in communication role-play using the components of active listening while performing a physical therapy intervention.
- Engage in nonverbal communication role-play contrasting open posture and closed posture situations while trying to establish a rapport with the patient.
- Observe and critique in the clinic the interaction between a PTA and a patient, recognizing effective and ineffective techniques.
- Compare and contrast in the clinic a SOAP progress note with a SOAP initial examination and evaluation report.
- Write a HEP describing the principles of proper body mechanics.
- Prepare and present a 15-minute presentation about communication methods for patients from other cultures.
- Perform three role-play situations using empathy, sympathy, and pity. Create a student panel to examine and contrast all three role-play situations.
- Interview a PT in private practice about his or her opinion of insurance reimbursement. Give a class presentation about the interview.
- Write a paper about insurance reimbursement in physical therapy.
- Critique a research article in class.

Communication Basics

CHAPTER

8

LEARNING OBJECTIVES

After studying Chapter 8, the reader will be able to:

- Discuss the role of therapeutic communication in physical therapy.
- Contrast empathy and sympathy.
- Describe the significance of verbal and nonverbal communication.
- Differentiate between verbal and nonverbal communication skills.
- Identify the elements required to establish a therapeutic relationship with the patient.
- List the seven kinds of listening skills and their importance to physical therapy.
- Discuss effective listening skills.
- Contrast open and closed postures.
- Describe written communication.
- Name the primary purpose of the home exercise program (HEP) handout.
- Describe the main elements of the home exercise program (HEP).

GLOSSARY

Ethnocentrism: The universal tendency of human beings to think that their ways of thinking, acting, and believing are the only right, proper, and natural ways; universal phenomena in that most people tend to believe that their ways of living, believing, and acting are right, proper, and morally correct.

Treatment plan: The projected series and sequence of treatment procedures based on an individualized evaluation of what is needed to restore or improve the health and function of a patient in physical therapy, the treatment plan gives direction to the medical care and provides an approach to measure the effectiveness of treatment.

Notes

CHAPTER 8

COMMUNICATION BASICS

Therapeutic Communication

- Therapeutic/healing manner
- Inner feelings, ideas, emotions, action between provider/patient
- Provider's total focus on patient
- Provider's objective listening to patient
- Trusting relationship provider/patient– provider's expertise and confidentiality–not parental role

---

Empathy

- Empathy: complete therapeutic partnership provider/patient–3 stages
- Listening to patient
- Provider lives patient's experience momentarily
- Provider/patient develop special alliance
- Self-awareness
- Contributes empathy development
- Starts around 2 years of age
- Helps recall own emotions
- Helps identify others' emotions
- Contributes morality development

Empathy

- ☐ Absence of empathy
  - People exploit/abuse others
  - Emotional/cognitive immaturity
  - Inability to love or relate others
  - Inability to respect/accept others' needs, feelings, hopes, choices, fears
- ☐ Empathy is different than sympathy–appropriate
- ☐ Pity is sympathy with condescension–inappropriate

Therapeutic Relationship

- ☐ Greet patient at eye level using patient's last name/title–cultural sensitivity
- ☐ Introduce: using name/title–inform patient of initial plan, advise patient of options, interventions
- ☐ Obtain patient's informed consent to treat
- ☐ Advise treatment's effects, indications, contraindications, alternatives
- ☐ Determine patient's participation during and after treatment
- ☐ Respond to patient's questions/concerns–promote patient's autonomy/responsibility

Verbal Communication

- ☐ Purposes
  - Establish rapport with patient
  - Obtain patient's information: condition and progress
  - Transmit pertinent information: others
  - Patient/patient family education
- ☐ Verbal communication problems
  - Ethnocentrism
  - Decreased cultural competence
  - Use family/friends as interpreters
  - Not use key words patient's language
  - Not use correct patient's last name

Verbal Communication in Physical Therapy Interventions

- ❑ **Successful communication in interventions**
- • **Focus patient's attention**
- • **Use simple, layperson's terms**
- • **General sequence prior to treatment**
- • **Patient's feedback before/during treatment**
- • **Clear, moderate tones, vary tone of voice**
- • **Sensitivity to patient's cultural background**
- ❑ **Effective listening methods**
- • **Patient free to talk—do not interrupt**
- • **Attention to patient's gestures, tone of voice, facial expressions, body posture**
- • **PTA clarifies, takes notes, reflects, shows involvement, empathizes**

Nonverbal Communication in Physical Therapy Intervention

- ❑ **Body language: postures, gestures, facial expressions, eye contact**
- • **Open posture: receives message, straight arms at sides, legs uncrossed**
- • **Closed posture: does not receive message, arms/legs crossed, body turned away**
- • **Acceptance thoughts: smiling, nodding**
- • **Rejection thoughts: eyes rolling, frowning**
- • **Unacceptable position: PTA stands and patient sits— PTA/patient same eye level**
- • **Eye contact (not staring): honesty, decision making capability**
- • **Touch: relaxing, caring, shows dedication, correct performance—use caution/consideration**

Physical Therapy Written Communication

- ❑ **Medical records**
- ❑ **Patient/patient family written instruction**
- ❑ **Informed consent**
- ❑ **Surveys**
- ❑ **Home exercise program handout**
- • **Organized and concise: few layman terms**
- • **Repetitions, resistance, positions**
- • **Diagrams and pictures: sorted logical manner, simple, PT/PTA contact information**
- • **Consistent clinical demonstrations**
- • **Treatment plan extension: starts first day treatment—written 5th grade level**

Documentation and the Medical Record

LEARNING OBJECTIVES

After studying Chapter 9, the reader will be able to:

- Describe the significance and the purpose of the physical therapy medical record.
- Identify the American Physical Therapy Association's (APTA's) guidelines in regard to physical therapy documentation.
- Discuss documentation elements of the initial examination (including the patient history), daily/weekly reports, progress reports, and discharge reports.
- Define the SOAP mnemonic and its meaning.

GLOSSARY

Assessment data: Data that include an appraisal or evaluation of a patient's condition based on clinical and laboratory data, medical history, and the patient's accounts of symptoms; data included in the "A" section of the SOAP note; in the SOAP note, they provide the rationale for the necessity of the skilled physical therapy services, interprets the data, and gives meaning to the data.

Disability: The inability to engage in age-specific, gender-related, and sex-specific roles in a particular social context and physical environment; it is also any restriction or lack (resulting from an injury) of ability to perform an activity in a manner or within the range considered normal for a human being.

Documentation data: All information related to patient's reasons for seeking medical care and patient's response to the medical care provided.

Medical diagnosis: Physician's identification of the cause of the patient's illness or discomfort.

Objective data: Data included in the "O" section of the SOAP note; they include information gathered by the health care provider through examination or assessment (or reassessment) of the patient; in the SOAP note are information that can be observed, measured, or reproduced by another health care provider with the same training as the initial provider.

Subjective data: Data included in the "S" section of the SOAP note; they include information gathered through an interview of the patient or a representative of the patient; all information gathered by the health care provider.

Treatment plan: The projected series and sequence of treatment procedures based on an individualized evaluation of what is needed to restore or improve the health and function of a patient in physical therapy, the treatment plan gives direction to the medical care and provides an approach to measure the effectiveness of treatment.

Notes

CHAPTER 9

**DOCUMENTATION AND
THE MEDICAL RECORD**

Medical Records

- ☐ **Purposes**
- • **Reimbursement**
- • **Quality care**
- • **Continuity of care**
- • **Legal: education**
- • **Research: marketing**
- ☐ **Types of records**
- • **POMR: data base, problem list, treatment plan, progress notes, discharge notes**
- • **SOMR: sections**
- • **SOAP**

APTA's Documentation Guidelines

- ☐ **Consistent APTA's Standards of Practice**
- ☐ **Legible: Approved abbreviations/symbols**
- ☐ **Black/blue ink: cross out mistakes, initial and date, record all communications**
- ☐ **Patient's name/number each page**
- ☐ **Include informed consent for each session**
- ☐ **Sign/date therapist's first and last name and designation**
- ☐ **PTA students' notes: cosigned PTA**
- ☐ **PT students and non-licensed notes: cosigned PT**

Physical Therapy Documentation Reports

- ☐ Initial examination and evaluation report
- • Foundation all other reports
- • Written PT
- • Written in SOAP, POMR, FOR formats
- ☐ Daily/weekly notes
- • Written PT/PTA
- ☐ Progress reports
- • Written PT
- • Continuum of care documentation
- ☐ Discharge reports
- • Written PT (as per APTA)

Daily/Weekly SOAP Format Notes

- ☐ S-Subjective data
- • Patient's/patient's family information
- • Patient own response to prior treatment, description of functional improvements
- • Patient complaints of pain: Lifestyle situations
- • Patient own goals: Compliance/difficulties HEP
- ☐ O-Objective data
- • Physical therapy measurements/tests
- • Description interventions/patient function
- • PT/PTA objective observations: increase reps., patient education/instruction

Daily/Weekly SOAP Format Notes

- ☐ A-Assessment data
- • Summary Subjective and Objective
- • PT/PTA assessment patient response and effectiveness treatment
- • PTA assessment patient progress STGs/LTGs
- • Reasons interventions
- • Interventions' effects on patient's impairments and functional limitations
- ☐ P-Plan data
- • Written future tense: "will increase reps."
- • PTA plan next session: "will add ex."
- • PTA plan: need PT re-examination or PT discharge

Legal Issues

- Comply: jurisdictional, regulatory, insurance requirements
- Patient's rights privacy
- Patient's authorization: release medical information
- Medical information inquiries: PT directed
- Physical therapy records: locked safe/secure place for 7 years

Telephone Referral Requirements

- Date/time call
- Name person called
- Name person took referral
- Name patient and referral details
- Date written copy referral
- Name PT: examine/evaluate referred patient

Notes

Teaching, Learning, and Medical Terminology

LEARNING OBJECTIVES

After studying Chapter 10, the reader will be able to:

- Discuss the teaching and learning aspects of physical therapy.
- Describe patient education methods for people who have difficulty reading, for patients who are older adults, for patients who have visual and hearing impairments, for patients who cannot speak English, and for patients from other cultures.
- Define medical terminology and its role in physical therapy.
- List the standardized terminology used in physical therapy.

Notes

CHAPTER 10

TEACHING, LEARNING, AND MEDICAL TERMINOLOGY

Clinical Instruction

- ☐ **Modes**
- · **Discussions/demonstrations**
- · **Presentations/lectures**
- · **Videotape/DVD: Return demonstrations**
- · **Illustrations/written information**
- ☐ **PT/PTA responsibilities**
- · **Gain learner attention: clear objectives**
- · **Recall prior: relate present to future learning–break down learning units/steps**
- · **Sequence: practice, progress comfort pace, feedback–knowledge results**
- · **Reward success: no negativity, fear, frustration, failure**

Four Learning Styles

- ☐ **Visual: symbols, charts, diagrams**
- · **Use mind mapping: visual aids, imaging techniques, no visual distractions**
- ☐ **Auditory, hear lectures: discuss topic**
- · **Use study groups, take lecture notes, tape lectures, quiet study**
- ☐ **Kinesthetic: "doing"–lab/clinical**
- · **Read material; use illustrations, case studies, write practice answers**
- ☐ **Analytic: read/think/organize–detail**
- · **See "big picture": organize material–no detail–not stuck on one concept**

Strategies for Improving Learning Skills

- ☐ Supportive relationships
- ☐ Expand personal learning style
- ☐ Study groups
- ☐ Improve match learning style and life
- • Change career, reorganize priorities: use learning style strengths/weaknesses
- ☐ Flexible learner
- • Long-term plan, long-term payoffs
- • Practice new skills, no punishment failure
- • Reward self

Test Exam Strategies

- ☐ Answer items student knows: skip others
- ☐ Focus on skipped items: eliminate incorrect answers
- ☐ Think critically
- • Cautious items: "always", "never", "invariably", "none", "all", "every", "must"
- • Substitute qualified term for absolute term: statement more/less valid than original

General Tips for Teachers and Learners

- ☐ Learner: sets own goals, freely expresses ideas/beliefs/concerns
- ☐ Teacher does not dictate learning
- ☐ Respect/trust: learner/teacher
- ☐ Teacher: supportive/nonjudgmental
- ☐ PT/PTA: academic/clinical teacher
- • Individuals learn at different rates
- • Learning: trial, error, introspection
- • Effective experiential learning
- • Learner reinforcement: competence and success

Patient Education Requirements

- Adapt teaching to patient learning
- Communicate clearly and simply use everyday words, use audio tapes and web sites
- Verify patient understanding: open-ended questions and demonstrations
- Patient–difficulty reading: use plain language, short and simple sentences, same words
- Patient–older adult: quiet place, sit near patient, brief sessions, speak clearly, practice each step, include patient family member or friend

Patient Education Requirements

- Patient with visual impairments
  - PT/PTA introduce themselves/other people room, ask if patient needs assistance
  - Use large print size, no italics, use Braille
  - Close to patient: light, get patient attention, speak clear and distinct (not loud)
  - Not exaggerated pronunciation
- Patient cannot speak English: certified interpreters, PT/PTA greet patient in native language, pronounce patient name correctly
- Patient from another culture: cultural competence, creative treatment

Medical Terminology and APTA Standardized Terminology

- Medical terminology
  - Latin and Greek terms
  - Prefix: word fragment–front–basic word
  - Suffix: word fragment–end–basic word
- APTA standardized terminology
  - PT/PTA: highest earned physical therapy degree–other earned academic degree–specialist certification–other degree/honor
  - SPT/SPTA
  - PT: professional
  - PTA: technically educated healthcare provider

Reimbursement and Research

LEARNING OBJECTIVES

After studying Chapter 11, the reader will be able to:

- Describe reimbursement for Medicare, Medicaid, private insurance companies, and health maintenance organizations.
- Discuss the main elements of research study, and describe how to write a research report.

GLOSSARY

Disability: The inability to engage in age-specific, gender-related, and sex-specific roles in a particular social context and physical environment; it is also any restriction or lack (resulting from an injury) of ability to perform an activity in a manner or within the range considered normal for a human being.

Notes

CHAPTER 11

REIMBURSEMENT AND RESEARCH

Reimbursement Terminology

- **First-party: patient**
- **Second-party: PT**
- **Third-party and payer: insurance**
- **Fee-for-service: fee each procedure**
- **Capitation: a set-fee payment**
- **Co-payment: patient payment portion**
- **Deductible: patient payment portion prior to insurance payments**
- **Denial: insurance refusal payment**
- **Eligibility: qualification (or not) insurance benefits**

Reimbursement Organizations

- **Medicare, established 1965**
  - **Administered: Center for Medicare and Medicaid Services (CMS)**
  - **Fee-for-service and HMO**
- **Medicaid, established 1965**
  - **Federal and state**
- **Private companies**
  - **Insurance, commercial, self-insured, indemnity plans, and private**
- **Health Maintenance Organization (HMO): managed care**

Medicare

- ☐ **Eligibility**
  - **Persons 65 years old or older**
  - **Persons under 65: long-term disability**
  - **Persons under 65: chronic renal disease**
  - **Widows 50 or older: eligible disability**
- ☐ **Part A–hospital insurance–physical therapy**
  - **Inpatient hospital and SNF**
  - **Certain HHA and hospice**
- ☐ **Part B–medical insurance–physical therapy**
  - **Outpatient and certain HHA**
  - **Durable medical equipment**
  - **20% co-payment**

Medicaid

- ☐ **Medicaid**
  - **Low-income families with children**
  - **Older individuals–blind–disability–Supplemental Security Income**
  - **Certain low-income pregnant women and children**
  - **Certain people–very high medical bills**
  - **Physical therapy–optional**
  - **Independent PT–Medicaid provider number**

Types of Research

- ☐ **Experimental–independent variable controlled manipulation by researcher**
  - **True/quasi experimental**
  - **Single subject–within subject and between subject design**
- ☐ **Nonexperimental–no manipulation independent variable**
  - **Case reports and correlational studies**
  - **Developmental and historical**
  - **Qualitative–action–case study–ethnography**

Physical Therapy Research Purposes

- ❑ Physical therapy research purposes
- • Establish profession body of knowledge
- • Determine efficacy interventions and improve patient care

Elements of a Research Study

- ❑ Elements of a research study
- • Title–informative, learn content
- • Abstract–specific concise overview
- • Introduction–motivation, detailed overview
- • Methods–subjects–design–instruments–data collection–data analysis
- • Results–findings
- • Discussion and Conclusion–interpretation results

Elements Used in Research

- ❑ Independent variable–researcher manipulated–brings change in dependent
- ❑ Dependent variable–effects of independent– determined outcome
- ❑ Research question–contributes scientific knowledge
- ❑ Reliability–intrarater and interrater
- ❑ Validity–internal and external
- ❑ Subjects–human, voluntary informed consent

Notes

PATIENT CARE ESSENTIALS FOR THE PHYSICAL THERAPIST ASSISTANT

PART

V

INTRODUCTION TO PART V

Part V of this text includes the following three chapters:

- Chapter 12: Infection Control, Patient Preparation, and Vital Signs
- Chapter 13: Patient Positioning, Body Mechanics, and Transfer Techniques
- Chapter 14: Wheelchairs, Assistive Devices, and Gait Training

The physical therapist (PT) and the physical therapist assistant (PTA) have complex and varied responsibilities during clinical practice. Some of these responsibilities may change depending on the type of clinical facility. For example, working in an outpatient orthopedic physical therapy department may require treating patients who in the majority would present with musculoskeletal disorders. In this orthopedic environment, the PT or the PTA may not be involved with elements of patient care such as positioning or transfers. Gait training may be taught on occasion to patients who postoperatively need to learn how to use crutches or walkers. In contrast, when working in a skilled nursing facility or in an inpatient hospital department, the PT and the PTA would almost constantly need to use positioning, transfers, gait training, wheelchair measurements, assistive devices, and other factors significant to patient care. Considering the variety of clinical practices, PTA students should become familiar early in their technical education with the varied elements of patient care. These should include vital signs, area and patient preparation, patient positioning, body mechanics and transfers, hand washing and infection control, wheelchair features, and gait training.

LABORATORY ACTIVITIES FOR PART V

The following activities are suggested to the instructor to involve students in the application of laboratory performances:

- Describe and demonstrate assessing vital signs.
- Role-play the therapist and patient by preparing the area for the patient's arrival, draping the patient prior to treatment, and establishing a therapeutic relationship with the patient.
- Demonstrate positioning for a patient with hemiplegia.
- Perform lifting techniques using the "five Ls."
- List and demonstrate bed mobility transfers.
- List and demonstrate sitting and standing transfers including the sliding board transfer.
- Practice hand washing for medical asepsis. Watch and critique another student's hand-washing technique.
- Give a class presentation describing the components of a wheelchair.
- Participate in a wheelchair training session at the local hospital.

- Working in groups of two, perform wheelchair measurements.
- Practice wheelchair training activities indoors.
- Analyze a classmate's subphases of gait and identify the major muscle groups involved in each subphase.
- Describe different types of assistive devices and perform the necessary measurements.
- Practice gait training using different assistive devices and gait sequencing patterns; practice on even surfaces and stairs.
- Perform guarding techniques on even surfaces and stairs.
- Demonstrate getting up with crutches or a walker from a wheelchair.

Infection Control, Patient Preparation, and Vital Signs

LEARNING OBJECTIVES

After studying Chapter 12, the reader will be able to:

- Employ proper hand washing and infection control techniques.
- Prepare the treatment area.
- Prepare the patient for treatment.
- Describe and assess blood pressure, pulse, respiration, and temperature.

GLOSSARY

Anemia: A condition in which there is a reduction in the number of red blood cells or hemoglobin in the bloodstream; the patient having anemia may exhibit generalized weakness and paleness.

Arteriosclerosis: Thickening and hardening of the arteries.

Asepsis: A condition free from germs, infections, and any form of living organism.

Dyspnea: Inability or difficulty breathing (shortness of breath).

Foley catheter: A urinary tract catheter with a balloon attachment at one end.

Hypertension: Any abnormally high blood pressure; blood pressure above 120/80.

Renal dialysis: The process of diffusing blood across a semipermeable membrane to remove toxic materials and to maintain fluid, electrolyte, and acid–base balance in cases of impaired kidney function or absence of the kidneys.

Vasodilation: Increase in the diameter of blood vessels, which increases blood flow.

Notes

CHAPTER 12

INFECTION CONTROL, PATIENT PREPARATION, AND VITAL SIGNS

Hand Washing

- ☐ Hand washing
  - Purpose: decrease number of germs on hands, infection control (sepsis prevention)
  - After touching blood, body fluids, secretions, wounds, dressings, bed linen, protective clothing
  - Before/after eating and toileting
  - After sneezing, coughing, nose blowing, removing gloves
  - Routine: plain soap for 30 seconds; infections: antiseptic agent for 60 seconds to 2 minutes

Hand Washing Procedures

- ☐ Remove jewelry: turn on mixed hot/cold water, wet hands and wrists, apply soap
- ☐ Use friction and circular motion, wash palms and backs each hand for 10 seconds each
- ☐ Interlace fingers: wash interspaces for 10 seconds each and wash wrist/lower forearm
- ☐ Use soft brush finger creases, cuticles, and under fingernails
- ☐ Rinse arms and hands, do not touch sink
- ☐ Dry hands, disposable paper towel (ready prior to washing), turn off faucets with paper towel

Microorganisms
Nosocomial Infections

☐ **Microorganisms**
- **Viruses and bacteria**
- **Fungi, protozoans, or intercellular parasites**

☐ **Nosocomial infections: hospital and hospital-like settings**
- **Pathoge: staphylococci, enterococci**
- **HostsL patients, compromised immune system**
- **Transmission: skin-to-skin, airborne, water, food, soil, animal sources**
- **Nosocomial infections: UTI, RTI, blood stream, surgical site, skin, gastrointestinal, CNS, fungal, pneumonia, MRSA, VRE**

CDC Guidelines
Infection Control

☐ **Use gloves when touching: blood, bodily fluids, secretions, excretions, contaminated items**

☐ **Apply clean gloves touching mucous membranes and nonintact skin**

☐ **Change gloves between tasks on same patient: high concentration microorganisms**

☐ **Wash hands immediately after glove removal**

☐ **Remove soiled gown after use and wash hands**

☐ **Soiled patient care equipment: do not touch skin and mucous membranes, clean and reprocess or discard single-use items**

CDC Guidelines
Infection Control

☐ **Airborne: tuberculosis, measles, chickenpox**
- **Respiratory isolation room–limit patient movement outside**
- **PTA mask–patient mask outside room**

☐ **Coughing, sneezing, talking–mumps, rubella, flu, pertussis**
- **Isolation room–limit patient movement outside**
- **PTA mask–patient mask outside room**

☐ **Direct patient contact–hand or skin-to-skin**
- **Isolation room–PTA gloves and gowns–touching patient/environment–limit patient movement**
- **Single-patient use equipment**

Area Preparation

- ☐ Last PT/PTA who used equipment
- • Returns equipment to storage
- • Ensures equipment functions properly
- • Cleans area to be ready for next patient
- ☐ Treatment area
- • Free of clutter
- • Open access transfer/gait
- • Necessary equipment prior treatment: supplies–ultrasound gel or massage oil, linens, towels or sheets

Physical Therapy Risk Management Procedures

- ☐ Maintenance/calibration twice a year–electrical equipment
- ☐ Staff education/training–use equipment safely
- ☐ Emergency cart–emergency situations, check daily supplies
- ☐ Equipment cleaning–whirlpool use bleach, povidone-iodine, Chloramine-T
- ☐ Report accidents
- ☐ Identify all risk factors–apply proper measures

Patient Preparation

- ☐ Hospital/SNF nursing staff prepares patient
- • PT/PTA notify nursing ahead
- • Patient dressed properly: shoes, 2 gowns, slacks, shorts
- • PT/PTA: not disrupt vital medical equipment ICU/CCU nurse–removes suction/feeding tubes–invasive monitoring
- • Transfer/gait training: Foley catheter–below bladder–2 inches above floor–repositioned
- ☐ Draping, prior treatment
- • Expose area–protect patient modesty
- • Patient comfort–not soil patient skin/clothing

Notes

Draping Procedures

- Patient consent: explain procedure
- Position patient: supine, sidelying, or prone
- Patient permission/reason disrobe: treatment gown, linens to cover
- Privacy: patient undressing, storage for patient clothes and valuable items
- Drape area to be treated: tuck in/tape linens not tightly
- Treatment: patient comfortable
- After treatment: remove draping, clean area
- Privacy: patient dressing street clothes and valuable items
- Dispose used linens: use proper container, prepare treatment area for next patient

Vital Signs

- BP
  - Systolic: heart contracting–healthy people– 90 mmHg and 120 mmHg
  - Diastolic: heart relaxes–healthy people– 60 mmHg and 80 mmHg
  - Hypertension: above 120/80 mmHg
  - Infants: low BP–80/50 mmHg, children low BP - 100/55 mmHg
  - BP increases proportional exercises/activities
  - Instruments: stethoscope, sphygmomanometer, BP cuff (wide for adults, narrow for infants and children)
  - Assess: typical–brachial artery

Procedures Taking BP

- PTA washes hands, gets patient consent, takes BP same arm
- Patient relaxed, arm horizontal at heart level
- BP cuff appropriate width/length
- Deflated BP cuff, position evenly and snugly on upper arm, 1–2 inches above antecubital fossa, close BP cuff valve
- Diaphragm stethoscope, brachial artery, sphygmomanometer zero
- Inflate BP cuff to 30 mmHg above patient normal BP prior readings
- Deflate BP cuff slowly, 2–3 mmHg
- First sound heard–systolic pressure, no longer sounds heard–diastolic pressure

Vital Signs

- ☐ **Pulse**
- **Rhythmical throbbing artery–result each heartbeat**
- **Normal adult: 70 bpm (60 bpm–100bpm)**
- **Normal: infant 120 bpm; child 125 bpm**
- **Bradycardia > 60 bpm**
- **Tachycardia < 100 bpm**
- **Routine: radial artery (base of thumb)**
- **Cardiac arrest: carotid artery–one side at a time, femoral artery**
- **Infant–carotid/brachial artery**
- **Lower extremity–popliteal/dorsalis pedis artery**

Vital Signs

- ☐ **Respiration**
- **Inhalation O2 to lungs–diaphragm and intercoastal muscles contract**
- **Exhalation CO2 from lungs–muscle relax**
- **Normal adult: 12 br/min–18 br/min**
- **Normal: infant 30 br/min; child 20 br/min**
- **Tachypnea: increased adult 20 br/min or more**
- **Bradypnea: decreased adult 10 br/min or less**
- ☐ **Temperature**
- **Normal adult: 98.6°F (37°C)**
- **If elevated: infectious conditions**

Procedures Taking Pulse/Respiration

- ☐ **PTA washes hands: second hand watch, paper and pencil, record data**
- ☐ **Patient consent take pulse: not aware assess respiration, altered rate**
- ☐ **Patient comfort/one arm across chest: respiration assessment**
- ☐ **PTA three fingers squarely/firmly (not too hard) over pulse site: not PTA thumb**
- ☐ **PTA watches patient arm across chest: counts inspirations 30 seconds x 2 and records**
- ☐ **Counts pulse 30 seconds x 2: cardiac dysfunctions, counts pulse 60 seconds and records**

Patient Positioning, Body Mechanics, and Transfer Techniques

LEARNING OBJECTIVES

After studying Chapter 13, the reader will be able to:

- Position the patient for treatment and to prevent pressure ulcers.
- Use proper body mechanics during patient's transfer or ambulation.
- Perform different types of bed mobility with patients
- Perform sitting transfers, and standing transfers with patients.

GLOSSARY

Decubitus ulcers: Open sores due to lowered circulation.

Hemiplegia: Condition in which half of the body is paralyzed; paralysis.

Joint contracture: Shortening of muscle and connective tissue limiting the range of motion at a joint.

Notes

CHAPTER 13

PATIENT POSITIONING, BODY MECHANICS, AND TRANSFER TECHNIQUES

Patient Positioning

- ☐ Prevent pressure ulcers (decubitus ulcers)
- Patient confined to bed: turn every 2 hours
- Patient confined chair: relieve pressure on buttocks every 15 minutes with push-ups or leaning forward/side-to-side
- Patient confined chair : sensory deficits, poor circulation, frail skin, relieve pressure on buttocks every 10 minutes
- Patients hemiplegia/amputations: special positioning techniques

---

Positioning Supine

- ☐ Bony prominences at risk: supine
- Occipital tuberosity
- Medial epicondyle humerus
- Spine/inferior angle scapula
- Vertebral spinous process, posterior iliac crest
- Sacrum, greater trochanter, head fibula
- Lateral malleolus, posterior calcaneus
- ☐ Positioning supine, face upward
- Cervical roll or small pillow under head
- Small pillow under popliteal areas and/or knees
- Rolled towel under ankles

Positioning Sidelying

- ☐ **Bony prominences at risk: sidelying**
- • **Lateral ear/ribs/acromion process**
- • **Lateral head humerus, Medial/lateral epicondyle humerus**
- • **Greater trochanter, medial/lateral femoral condyles, tibial/fibular malleolus**
- ☐ **Positioning sidelying**
- • **1 to 2 pillows under head**
- • **Uppermost upper limb: pillow hold–not roll forward**
- • **Uppermost lower limb: slightly forward–1 or 2 pillows between knees and lower leg**
- • **Lowermost lower limb: slightly backward**

Positioning Prone

- ☐ **Bony prominences at risk: prone**
- • **Forehead, lateral ear, tip acromion process**
- • **Anterior head humerus, sternum, anterosuperior iliac spine, patella**
- • **Tibial ridge, dorsum foot**
- ☐ **Positioning prone, horizontal face downward**
- • **1 pillow under head or table face cutout**
- • **1 pillow under lower abdomen: decrease lumbar lordosis**
- • **Rolled towel under each anterior shoulder: elbows bent at 90 degrees in T position**
- • **Pillow under anterior ankles**

Positioning Sitting

- ☐ **Bony prominences at risk: sitting**
- • **Scapula**
- • **Vertebral spinous processes**
- • **Ischial tuberosities**
- ☐ **Positioning sitting**
- • **Feet: footstool, WC footrest**
- • **Hips/knees: 90 degrees flexion**
- • **Ankles: neutral**

Lifting Techniques

- ❑ **Wide BOS: feet wide anterior-posterior stance, stability**
- ❑ **PTA COG: anterior S2 vertebra, close to patient COG, decreased energy expenditure**
- ❑ **Five Ls in lifting**
- • **Load: appropriate weight**
- • **Lever: weight close to PT/PTA body, combined COG within same BOS**
- • **Lordosis: normal posture/lordotic curve**
- • **Legs: large muscle groups**
- • **Lungs: exhale while lifting**

General Transfer Techniques

- ❑ **Preparation for transfer**
- • **Read patient chart: medical/physical therapy diagnosis, medical history**
- • **Current level of function: POC (STGs and LTGs)**
- • **Prior treatment, last assessment: MD/SW/RN**
- ❑ **General transfer principles**
- • **Plan transfer: obtain patient consent and cooperation**
- • **Acquire and check equipment**
- • **Prepare patient for transfer: secure area/transfer surface**
- • **Position surface: use proper body mechanics**

General Transfer Techniques

- ❑ **Safety belt**
- • **Patient safety: stability, control do not hold on to patient clothing/shoulder/wrist**
- • **Risk management control: PT/PTA/patient safety, facility liability control**
- ❑ **Types physical therapy assistance**
- • **Minimal Assist: PTA 25% total patient work**
- • **Moderate Assist: PTA 50% total patient work**
- • **Maximum Assist: PTA 75% total patient work**
- • **Independent: PTA supervises**
- • **CGA: constant guarding, SGA: intermittent guarding, SBA: ready give light assist**

Notes

Types of Transfers

- ☐ Bed mobility transfers–patient turning in bed
- · Independent
- · Assisted
- ☐ Sitting transfers
- · Assisted–sliding board
- · Independent
- · Dependent lift: one or two PTAs, draw sheet, zero lifting: power/manual lifts
- ☐ Standing transfers
- · Assisted pivot
- · Independent pivot
- · Standby pivot

Sliding Board Transfer Procedures

- ☐ PTA obtains: safety belt, WC, sliding board, gets patient consent, explains procedure to patient
- ☐ WC 45 degrees bed: adjust surfaces WC/bed
- ☐ Remove WC armrest/footrest near bed, safety belt patient
- ☐ Sliding board one side under patient buttocks/thighs, other side WC seat
- ☐ PTA guards/instructs patient not catch fingers under sliding board
- ☐ Patient push ups sliding board, leaning slightly forward, completes transfer, positioned WC

Sitting Dependent Transfer Procedures

- ☐ PTA plans: safety belt, WC, gets patient consent, explains procedure to patient
- ☐ WC 45 degrees bed: remove WC armrest and footrest near bed, safety belt patient
- ☐ Folds patient arms in lap, slides patient EOB
- ☐ PTA wide BOS: braces patient's involved limb
- ☐ PTA bends patient trunk, head on PTA hip
- ☐ PTA lifts patient by safety belt, on each side
- ☐ PTA moves feet, slowly lowers patient WC
- ☐ PTA positions patient comfortable in WC

Standing Assisted Pivot Transfer Procedures

- ☐ **PTA obtains safety belt, WC and patient consent**
- ☐ **PTA explains procedure patient, applies safety belt patient, WC 45 degrees bed**
- ☐ **PTA instructs: patient strong limb near WC–patient lock WC, elevate foot-plate, strong limb backward, weak limb forward**
- ☐ **PTA instructs: patient lean forward–place arm near WC on armrest, rock body back/forth, get momentum, stand**
- ☐ **PTA instructs: patient balance–switch armrests, patient pivot back toward WC, lower down slowly WC, patient position WC**

Notes

Wheelchairs, Assistive Devices, and Gait Training

LEARNING OBJECTIVES

After studying Chapter 14, the reader will be able to:

- Discuss the types of wheelchairs and wheelchair components.
- Measure the wheelchair for the patient.
- Identify wheelchair training techniques.
- Describe the two phases of human gait: the stance and the swing phase.
- List the types of assistive devices used in physical therapy.
- Explain and perform preambulatory activities at the parallel bars.
- Follow guarding techniques during ambulation on even surfaces and stairs.
- Discuss patients' weight-bearing categories.
- Differentiate between different weight-bearing categories such as non-weight bearing, partial weight bearing, toe touch weight bearing, and weight bearing as tolerated.
- List the six gait sequencing patterns used in gait training.
- Perform the six gait sequencing patterns using different assistive devices.
- Discuss standing and sitting activities using assistive devices.
- Describe ascending and descending stairs using crutches and the cane.

GLOSSARY

Hemiplegia: Condition in which half of the body is paralyzed; paralysis.

Notes

CHAPTER 14

WHEELCHAIRS, ASSISTIVE DEVICES, AND GAIT TRAINING

Wheelchairs

- ☐ WC Purposes
- Correct and straighten deformity
- Increase and maintain level of function
- Allow patient maximum functional use
- ☐ Proper WC seating/positioning
- Prevents deformity and pressure ulcers
- Normalizes tone
- Promotes efficient use of upper limbs
- Enhances respiratory function
- Body alignment
- Increases sitting comfort and tolerance

Wheelchair Types

- Standard: patients < 200 pounds
- Heavy duty: patients > 200 pounds
- Child: up to 6 years old, junior, adolescents, and smaller patients
- Amputation: bilateral limbs, drive wheels 2 inches back, WC not to tip backward
- Hemiplegia: 2 inches lower, propels with unaffected upper and lower limb
- One-arm drive: propels with one hand
- Tilt-in-space: tone/spasm hip/knee extensors, pressure relief
- Reclining: maintains upright sitting position
- Sport: plays sports
- Electric: joystick drive

Notes

Wheelchair Components and Measurements

- ☐ Seat, standard: sling
- • Seat width: widest part of hips plus 2 inches
- • Seat depth: posterior buttocks lateral thigh to popliteal fossa minus 2 inches
- • Seat height: floor bottom footplate = 2 inches
- ☐ Back, standard: sling
- • WC seat to lower angle scapula or shoulder top, depends on patient needs
- ☐ Two leg-rests, two footrests
- • Leg-length: bottom of shoe to under popliteal fossa minus 2 inches
- ☐ Armrests, WC frame, caster wheels, drive wheels, tires, brakes

Wheelchair Measurement Problems

- • Excessive seat width: difficult to reach drive wheels and maneuver tight places
- • Narrow seat width: pressure/discomfort
- • Short seat depth: no support on thighs
- • Long seat depth: less blood circulation to posterior knees
- • Low footplates: pelvis slides forward
- • High footplates: pressure to ischial tuberosities
- • Short leg length: pressure sores to ischial tuberosities
- • Long leg length: patient slides forward
- • High back: cannot reach projection hand, WC cannot fit in car

Wheelchair Training

- ☐ WC training: propulsion, level surfaces, doorways, elevators, uneven surfaces, curbs, stairs, falling safely
- • Wheelies: balance rear drive wheels
- • Ascend curb: caster wheels up on curb, push rear drive wheels using momentum
- • Descend curb: forward wheelie, backward leaning head/trunk forward
- • Fall forward: reach forward upper limbs, bend elbows, turn pelvis land on one hip
- • Fall backward: bend trunk/head reaching forward, fall on buttocks, protect head

Assistive Devices

□ **Roles**
- **Decreased strength to trunk and lower limbs**
- **Weight bearing restrictions**
- **Decreased functional mobility, stability, balance, coordination**
- **Increased pain during ambulation, neurological deficits, amputations, new orthotic and prosthetic devices**

Assistive Devices

□ **Types**
- **Canes: use outside clinic**
- **Crutches: use outside clinic**
- **Walkers, most stable: use outside clinic**
- **Parallel bars, most stable: use in clinic only**

Cane

□ **Cane**
- **Widens BOS, increases balance and stability, pain relief, does not reduce weight bearing**
- **Use opposite hand of affected lower limb**
- **Types: standard–wood or aluminum, use on stairs; quad, four point contact; hemi-walker**
- **Measurements–patient shoes: 6 inches lateral border of patient's toes; top of cane, greater trochanter; elbow flexed 20–30 degrees**
- **Gait sequences: simultaneous affected lower limb and cane, unaffected lower limb; cane: affected lower limb, unaffected lower limb**

Notes

Crutches

- ❑ Crutches
- Increase BOS, increase lateral stability
- Reduce weight bearing on lower limbs
- Awkward small areas: leaning creates damage radial nerve/axillary artery
- Made of wood and aluminum
- Types: auxiliary, standard, forearm
- Measurements–patient shoes: auxiliary, 2 inches bellow axilla to 6 inches in front and 2 inches lateral patient's foot; forearm, cuff at 1–1.5 inches below elbow
- Gait sequences: 2 point, 3 point, modified 3 point, 4 point, swing to, swing through

Walker

- ❑ Walker
- Provides wide BOS, increases anterior and lateral stability, easy to use
- Reduces weight bearing on lower limbs
- Cumbersome small spaces, no stairs
- Types: rigid, folding, rolling, reciprocal, stair climbing, hemi-walker
- Measurements: patient standing, shoes – elbow 20 – 30 degrees of flexion; top–greater trochanter
- Ambulate standard walker: lift walker forward, walker back legs same level patient's toes
- Gait sequences: 3 point, modified 3 point

Parallel Bars Training

- ❑ Patient guarding: front, slightly lateral to affected lower limb
- ❑ Balance activities
- Anterior/posterior/lateral weight shifts
- Hip hiking
- Stepping forward: shift weight backward
- ❑ Standing push-ups from WC
- ❑ Walking forward with appropriate weight bearing
- ❑ Turning toward unaffected lower limb: step small circles
- ❑ Walking forward using assistive device: turning

Guarding Techniques

- Level surfaces: posterior/lateral affected lower limb
- Ascending stairs: behind, slightly to side affected lower limb
- Descending stairs: front, slightly to side affected lower limb
- Key points of control
  - Shoulder and opposite pelvis
  - Safety belt
- Losing balance forward: PTA pulls patient by safety belt, holds patient anterior shoulder
- Losing balance backward: PTA holds safety belt, assists posterior shoulder, PTA lower limb assists pelvis

Gait Sequencing Patterns

- 4 point gait: slow, stable, weakness in lower limbs, WBAT/FWB–crutches or 2 canes
- 3 point gait: NWB gait, one affected lower extremity, patient good strength upper limbs, trunk, and unaffected lower limb, NWB/PWB/TTWB/WBAT–walker or crutches
- Modified 3 point gait: not strength/energy, WBAT/FWB–walker or crutches
- 2 point gait: closest to normal gait, FWB/PWB/TTWB/WBAT–crutches or 2 canes
- Swing to and swing through: paralysis both limbs, trunk instability–crutches

Weight Bearing Categories and Gait Sequences

- MD/DO establishes WB status
- NWB: 0% patient's weight, 3 point gait, assistive device advances simultaneously with affected limb
- PWB: toe touch to 20% to 50% patient's weight; TTWB: light touch patient's heel; 3 point gait and 2 point gait–assistive device advances simultaneously with affected limb
- WBAT: as much weight as tolerated–2 point, 3 point, modified 3 point, 4 point
- FWB: no weight bearing restrictions–2 point, 3 point, modified 3 point, 4 point

Notes

Ascending and Descending Stairs with Assistive Devices

- Ascending stairs: unaffected lower limb goes up first
- Descending stairs: affected lower limb goes down first
- Ascending/descending stairs: affected lower limb goes up/down together with assistive device
- PTA one foot: on step where patient stands, PTA other foot: on step below
- Assistive devices–stairs: standard cane, small-based quad cane, crutches